Health care in transition:
directions for the future

Health care in transition: directions for the future

by
Anne R. Somers

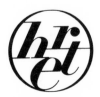

Hospital Research and Educational Trust
840 North Lake Shore Drive • Chicago, Illinois 60611

ISBN 0-87914-005-4
Library of Congress Catalog Card Number: 77-160033

HRET T-24
First printing 10M—5/71—165
Second printing 5M—11/71—200
Third printing 10M—3/72—221
Fourth printing 10M—8/73—280
Price: $3.95

For Mark Berke

These are times when we have to mold and to act, rather than be passive and react. . . . These are times when we must ourselves become change agents for society.

MARK BERKE
Presidential inaugural address,
American Hospital Association (1970)

It is said that we face a crisis in medicine today. . . . When the Chinese write the word "crisis," they do so in two characters, one meaning danger, the other, opportunity.

JOHN ROMANO, M.D.
Journal of the American Medical
Association (October 26, 1964)

Contents

Foreword

At no time in the history of the United States has there been greater need for informed opinion on the delivery of health care. The decisions on the organization and financing of health services that must be made today will affect us all for years to come. Mounting complexities and inequities, rising costs, and disparities in quality and distribution have posed problems that confront citizens in every walk of life, and bills embodying proposed solutions to those problems are proliferating in every legislative hall.

In this book, Anne Somers draws upon her years of study in the health care field to set forth the issues and alternatives. The book began with a study for the Board on Medicine of the National Academy of Sciences. Later, this was enlarged upon in a report prepared for the Governor's Steering Committee on Social Problems [New York]. That report was brought to the attention of the Hospital Research and Educational Trust, and it was agreed that the content met a long-felt need for a straightforward clarification of the basic elements in the organization and financing of health services, and should be made available to a wide audience. Accordingly, the manuscript was extensively revised in depth, and updated to the close of 1970, for this book.

We commend *Health Care in Transition* to all who are concerned about health care today, and who seek to contribute to the great debate that is now in progress.

EDWIN L. CROSBY, M.D.
Executive Vice President
Hospital Research and Educational Trust

Acknowledgments

I am grateful to many busy and knowledgeable individuals for their invaluable assistance. Those who reviewed all or parts of the manuscript in an earlier form include my husband, Herman M. Somers, and the following friends: Lynn Carmichael, M.D., President, The Society of Teachers of Family Medicine; Robert Cathcart, Vice President, Pennsylvania Hospital, Philadelphia, and Chairman, American Hospital Association Committee on Health Care for the Disadvantaged; Ward Darley, M.D., former Executive Director, Association of American Medical Colleges; James E. Hague, Associate Director and Editor-in-Chief, American Hospital Association; Susan S. Jenkins, Adviser to the Director, Bureau of Health Insurance, Social Security Administration; Marjorie M. Lawson, Director of Publications, Hospital Research and Educational Trust; George Melcher, M.D., President, Group Health Insurance, Inc.; Andrew E. Ruddock, Director, Bureau of Retirement, Insurance, and Occupational Health, U.S. Civil Service Commission; Steven Sieverts, Executive Director, Hospital Planning Association of Allegheny (Pa.) County; Robert M. Sigmond, Vice President for Planning, Albert Einstein Medical Center, Philadelphia; and Albert W. Snoke, M.D., Office of the Governor of Illinois, Chicago.

To David Kessner, M.D., Study Director, and Joseph Murtaugh, former Secretary, Board on Medicine, National Academy of Sciences, and to Victor Weingarten, Director, Governor Rockefeller's Steering Committee on Social Problems, I am indebted for encouragement of this undertaking at an earlier stage.

It goes without saying that none of these bears any responsibility for the final product.

A.R.S.

Princeton, New Jersey
October 1970

PART ONE

Four Paradoxes

I am assuming that the modern world is, in fact, as revolutionary as everybody
says it is. Its profound contradictions are not due to mere perversity or folly.
They are due to the extraordinary developments in science and technology, which
have led to far more rapid and radical change than any previous society has known,
and than our society has been prepared to deal with. And because the paradoxes
of our age are so violent, men have been violently oversimplifying its issues. On
the one hand, many political and business leaders are celebrating the triumphs of
technology, science, and free enterprise as if there were nothing fundamentally
wrong with our civilization, and the world depressions and world wars were un-
fortunate accidents. On the other hand, many intellectuals are ignoring the obvious
triumphs, seeing only a monstrous folly and evil. I have assumed that it might be
helpful to try viewing our world with both pride and alarm, both tempered by
historical sense.

HERBERT J. MULLER
The Uses of the Past (1952)

The proverbial visitor from another planet would surely be baffled by the violently
contradictory reports on medical care in the United States that characterize both
public and private discussion. So, too, are many Americans—both providers and
consumers of medical care.

On the one hand, attention is called to continual evidence of astounding progress: the discovery and application of cures, drugs, diagnostic and surgical techniques that can only be described as "miracles." Imaginative new health care delivery
programs, representing billions of dollars, have been inaugurated under both public
and private auspices. Some 20 million elderly persons now have protection against
at least the most expensive medical care. Several million additional indigent and
medically indigent are receiving noncharity medical care for the first time in their
lives. Twenty new medical schools have been started in the past decade, as have
many additional schools for other health professions. Quality controls and drug
testing are more rigorous than ever before.

On the other hand, there are constant allegations of inadequate medical care,
unfilled health needs, exorbitant rises in costs, galloping inflation, and apparently
widespread discontent with most medical institutions. Every national administration
since 1961 has emphasized the "crisis in health care," and prescriptions for dealing
with it have become national political issues. Some knowledgeable politicians as well
as health experts expect it to become *the* major domestic issue of the 1970s, perhaps
as early as the 1972 presidential election.

I have assumed, with Professor Muller, that it would be helpful to view the world of health care with "both pride and alarm, both tempered by historical sense." In this light the progress and the difficulties appear as reverse sides of the same coin— a series of frustrating but understandable paradoxes. The vast, difficult, and perplexing problems of the present are seen, in large part, as products of earlier and continuing progress. Frequently, they represent primarily the dislocations and the need for adjustment created by more rapid advance in one area of knowledge— usually science and technology—than in others—usually social and economic organization—with resulting tensions in the social fabric and in our moral and ethical value systems.

The purpose of this book is twofold: First, to point up some of the major historical trends in the health care field and to identify the principal unresolved issues that are contributing to the impending crisis. To do this, four crucial factors were selected: the changing physician, the changing patient, the changing hospital, and changing patterns in financing. These are the subjects of Part One, Chapters 1 through 4.

Second, despite the emphasis on history, there is no preordained determinism in this great human drama. The element of free choice, our responsibility for decision making, cannot be evaded. So Part Two, Chapters 5 through 8, attempts to indicate the general directions in which satisfactory solutions are most likely to be found. The words "general directions" need underscoring. They are guideposts only, not blueprints.

The relationship between Part One and Part Two is apparent. Health Education relates to the New Patient; Redefinition of Professional Roles to the New Physician; Rationalization of Community Health Services to the New Hospital; and National Health Insurance to New Developments in Financing.

Needless to say, in a book of this length, there has been no attempt to be all-inclusive. Today, "health problem" is virtually synonymous with the "problem of human existence." Industrialization, urbanization, education, environmental pollution, war, crime, racial problems, housing, city planning or the lack of it: all of these and many additional factors bear importantly on the health of the people. Indeed, some have greater influence than health care as generally understood. It is not a matter of priority but of simple organizational necessity that these other factors are not discussed. The subject of this book is personal health care.

Even in this narrower field, hard choices had to be made. Many important aspects are omitted. Those that are included, however—the doctor, the patient, the hospital, the financing mechanism—are the *sine qua non* of any modern health care system.

Chapter 1

THE PHYSICIAN

The bestowal of your doctorates marks your near approach but not yet your arrival at the half-way mark in the training that is to qualify you for the practice of medicine. By average current experience, you still have 4.3 years of internship, residency, and postgraduate fellowship to go. . . . Four and a half years from now you will each have mastered some branch, corner, or aspect of the technology of medicine, and you will have differentiated into one or another of an ever-increasing variety of specialists. From this it follows that the hallowed image of the one-to-one, face-to-face, physician-patient relationship no longer fits the reality of medical care.

GERARD PIEL
Commencement address,
Cornell University Medical College (1968)

What do we ask of ourselves? Practical cold questions such as: If I become an orthopedic surgeon will I be expected to take complete care of the patient—the glaucoma, the depression, the urinary tract infection—or should I see that others do? If I am a general practitioner should I try to do everything even if it makes me superficial? If I go into great depth in research or specialization how do I avoid waking up at age 45 plagued by questions of relevance in a society full of pieces that do not seem to fit together anymore? And if I manifest broad interests—tackle everything and worry about relevance—how do I avoid waking up at 45 plagued with the issue of effectiveness and spreading myself too thin?

LAWRENCE L. WEED, M.D.
Commencement address,
Case Western Reserve University School of Medicine (1969)

The Modern Miracle Worker

The typical modern doctor, with his specialized training, his hospital affiliation, and his access to the miraculous tools of modern technology and chemotherapy, is as different from the doctor of 50 years ago as the computer from the abacus, or the modern operating room from its 19th century predecessor. He can perform feats of surgery and diagnosis that stagger the imagination. He can, in some instances, literally raise the dead.

The lengthening life-span, the generally improved quality of life, and the ever-rising expectations with respect to health that characterize the modern patient (Chapter 2) are testimony to the increasing effectiveness of the modern physician as well as to progress in many other aspects of modern life—higher incomes, better

5

housing, better nutrition, better control of work hazards, etc. Perhaps the doctor has received more credit in this respect than he deserves. But in any case he is—to the general public—the symbol of progress in modern medicine and it is no wonder that he is in great demand.

His average age is 46.[1] He is very likely to be male (only seven percent of U.S. physicians are women) and white (only two percent are black).[2] He works long hours (63 a week in 1969), far longer than the average American worker although probably no longer than the average university professor, lawyer, or corporation executive.

The Bittersweet Fruits of Success

The modern doctor is well paid—the highest paid professional in the country. According to *Medical Economics,* the median self-employed physician netted $34,730 in 1967, ranging from $53,740 for neurosurgeons down to $27,600 for pediatricians. By 1969 the overall figure was $38,470.[3]

During the early post-World War II years physicians' fees, as measured by the U.S. Bureau of Labor Statistics' Consumer Price Index (CPI), rose less, on average, than the general cost of living. During the 1950s, the relationship was reversed; after 1965, dramatically so. From 1960 to 1965, the average annual rise for fees was 2.8 percent, compared to 1.3 percent for the general cost of living and 1.8 percent for all services except medical care. From 1968 to 1969, the corresponding figures were 7.0, 5.4, and 6.8, respectively. In the first quarter of 1970, doctors' fees rose 2.3 percent—an annual rate of 9.2 percent—compared to 1.4 percent for the overall CPI.

Practice costs are rising too. So are the hours of work and the number of patients seen per week. If one were to judge solely on the basis of scientific achievement, productivity, and income, one would have to conclude that "the doctor never had it so good."

But this is only one side of the coin. On the reverse are the negative aspects: the doctor shortage, the long hours, the unrelenting pressure on the profession as a whole and on the individual physician for more and better services, the rising costs of medical care, the alleged depersonalization of care, and the declining public image of the profession.

The Doctor Shortage

At first view, the allegations as to a physician shortage may appear exaggerated. There were, at the end of 1967, some 260,000 doctors—nonfederal doctors of medicine and osteopathy, including interns and residents—reported to be actually providing patient care either in their offices or as part of a hospital medical staff.[4] This is approximately 130 doctors per 100,000 civilian population, a ratio slightly greater than that four years earlier. In 1963 it was 124 per 100,000.

However, the apparent trend toward more doctors per capita is highly misleading as a guide to the adequacy of supply for a number of reasons, including the following:

[1]For this and succeeding notes in this chapter, see page 13.

1. **We are far too dependent on the importation of foreign-trained doctors.** An estimated 48,000 were in the United States as of Jan. 1, 1970.[5] The number now entering each year—estimates range from 8,000 to 10,000—is probably equal to the total output of all our medical schools. Most of the foreign graduates come for a few years only as hospital house staff, and the majority go home eventually. But many do not. Twenty-three percent of all doctors licensed in the United States in 1969 were foreign-trained.[6] This represents an increase of 50 percent over the yearly average of new foreign-trained licentiates for the previous 10-year period.

Aside from the doubtful ethics of this "brain-drain" of the underdeveloped areas, where most of the foreign physicians come from, and the questionable long-range reliability of the supply,[7] there is a serious question as to the training and competence of many. Their qualifications have undoubtedly improved in the past few years, thanks principally to the efforts of the Educational Council for Foreign Medical Graduates and its sponsors. Nevertheless, the pressure both from American hospitals and doctors for more house staff and from the graduates themselves for entry to the United States is so great that it is virtually impossible to maintain standards applicable to graduates of American medical schools.

2. **The geographic distribution of physicians is very uneven.** While New York had 199 MDs and DOs providing patient care per 100,000 population in 1967, Mississippi had only 69. The District of Columbia had 318 per 100,000, while many rural counties had none.

3. **The increasing proportion of specialists has further reduced the number of doctors available for general medical care.** An increasing proportion are not engaged in patient care at all but are spending all or most of their time in research, administration, teaching, government service, or consultation activities. Among those engaged primarily in patient care, the proportion in "primary care" has fallen dramatically.

According to the American Academy of General Practice, only 21 percent of United States physicians were in general practice in the spring of 1969.[8] Recent reports indicate that only 2 percent of medical students now in school are considering going into general practice and nearly half of the doctors now entering general practice were trained abroad. This situation will probably become even more extreme.

Moreover, the shortage applies not only to GPs but to all those who might be identified as "generalists" or engaged in family practice. In 1950, the ratio of family practitioners—GPs, internists, and pediatricians—to population was 76 per 100,000. By 1965, it was only 50 per 100,000.[9] It is undoubtedly even less today.

Establishment in February 1969 of the new specialty of "Family Medicine" with its own examining board should lead to a new and better trained breed of family specialists. Whether it will have any appreciable effect on the general physician-population ratio or even on the proportion of doctors in primary practice is not known.

Aside from the problem of primary physicians, the distribution of other physicians is not calculated to produce the most efficient results. For example, 27 percent of all doctors in the United States are full-time surgeons; only 8 percent in England.[10] Whether there is a shortage of surgeons in England is debatable—the waiting lists for elective surgery are reported to be long—but by the ultimate test of comparative mortality the British do better than we do and, in any case, the difference between 8 percent and 27 percent is so great as to suggest that some adjustment might be in order in both countries.

4. **Educational requirements for doctors are constantly rising.** Despite the efforts of a few medical schools to shorten the required curriculum, it is almost impossible for a doctor to start practice today without 9 to 11 years of education beyond high school. The residency requirements for specialty practice continue to lengthen. For example, the American College of Surgeons now requires four instead of three years of surgical residency. Thus, even the general surgeon now has to put in 12 years of training beyond high school plus two years of military service. He will be about 30 before he can be on his own. For most this will mean a maximum of 30 to 35 years of practice—not much more than the period of childhood and preparation. This is a very important factor in the supply and demand equation and in our rising medical costs.

We have created 20 new medical schools and spent hundreds of millions of federal, state, and philanthropic dollars during the past decade on expansion of medical education in our attempts to meet the growing shortage. There has been progress. There were 33 percent more medical students in 1966-67 than there were in 1949-50, compared with a 30 percent rise in civilian population.[11] But this is still nothing like enough to meet the continuing rise in demand for medical services (Chapter 2). Nor, if past experience is any guide, will it bring more doctors to those rural areas and big city ghettos which already have the lowest doctor-population ratios. Nor is there any evidence that it will mean any substantial rise in the number of primary doctors—the category in shortest supply today.

The American Medical Association, once opposed to increasing the number of doctors, is now in the forefront of those urging the need for more. "The No. 1 priority should be to increase the output and production of physicians," said Dr. W. C. Bornemeier, in his inaugural address as AMA president in 1970. There is a present shortage, he claimed, of 50,000, which will rise to 80,000 within the decade.[12]

Rising Productivity: Good or Bad?

Our apparent inability to correct the physician supply and demand imbalance has increased pressure for greater physician productivity. Here, too, progress has been made. Thirty years ago, the average doctor saw about 50 patients a week. Today he averages 132; the GP sees even more, 173.[13] This was made possible by many factors—more use of the telephone and the automobile and of nurses, technicians, and other health personnel, better organization of office practice, greater use of the hospital as a site for patient visits, the almost complete disappearance of the house call, and so forth.

Although the proportion of doctors working in *formal* group practices is still relatively small—about 11 percent in 1965[14]—the proportion in some form of combined practice—either hospital-based or office-based—is growing rapidly. According to the AMA, there were 59,194 nonfederal MDs working as full-time hospital staff, interns, residents, or fellows at the end of 1967.[15] Another 24,917 were working in the same capacities for the federal government. This means that about 31 percent of all doctors engaged in patient care were on hospital salary or stipends. If one adds to this *Medical Economics'* estimate of 39 percent of self-employed physicians working in partnership or some other form of nonsolo practice[16] (74,131), it appears that nearly 60 percent of actual patient care in the United States is being rendered by doctors engaged in some form of combined practice. This does not take into account the important and growing tendency of solo practitioners to locate their offices in a single building in, or adjacent to, a hospital. In many communities, the emphasis on "balanced tenancy" and the degree of informal cooperation between such doctors amounts to an elementary form of group, or at least grouped, practice.

The employment of allied health personnel increases, year by year. Some 3.5 to 4 million persons are now engaged in the many aspects of health services and this does not include the million or so engaged in the manufacture and wholesale distribution of drugs. This extensive complex, comprising about 375 job titles,[17] was already, in 1960, the nation's third largest industry and one of the two fastest growing. Projections indicate that either health services or education will soon be the nation's largest consumer of manpower. Within the great overall growth, perhaps the most striking single fact is the declining ratio of doctors to all health personnel. It is now in the order of 1 to 11.

Some experts believe this trend can, and should, be pushed still further. It has become fashionable to speak of the health services industry as a "cottage industry," the invidious reference applying primarily to the continued existence of the solo practitioner or the small partnership. The physician is constantly exhorted to make greater use of the computer, closed-circuit TV, and other technological aids, to delegate still more tasks to "paramedics," to form more and larger groups, and generally to take the lead in transforming the "cottage industry" into a "rational integrated health care system." The inference, it appears, is that the more patient visits, the more surgical or other procedures the physician can produce, the better our health will be.

Others feel that continued quantitative increases and greater systemization can only be at the expense of quality and are likely to lead to further deterioration in the doctor-patient relationship, and, possibly, in the national health. Some critics of present trends claim that the emphasis on physician productivity—usually measured as so many patient visits or procedures per day or per week—has already reached the point of superficiality, if not worse. A 1967 survey of Kentucky GPs by the University of Kentucky College of Medicine Department of Community Medicine reported the average length of time spent by the doctor with each patient as 6.1 minutes, with the median 4.7 minutes.[18]

The growing evidence of unnecessary prescribing, surgery, and other forms of treatment, especially for well-insured patients or those on Medicare or Medicaid, should be warning enough that quantitative increases alone constitute a highly inadequate and probably dangerous goal in this complex field. The strict economic definition of "productivity" incorporates the concept of quality; thus an increase in patient visits accompanied by poorer quality care should not be considered a "productivity increase." However, it is much easier to count the number of visits than to measure subtle changes in quality.

"Docs" and "Crocks" — The Widening Gap

Whatever the reason, or combination of reasons, it is clear that public dissatisfaction with the medical profession is conspicuously on the rise. To some extent this is part of the general decline in respect for authority—whether represented by parent, university president, or doctor. In part, it is the revolt of the young against the "Establishment." But in the case of the doctor there appears to be a special ingredient, aimed primarily at an apparent discrepancy between the ideal image of the selfless dedicated "father-priest-healer" figure of the past and the "cold scientific money-seeker" of the present. Also, of course, the degree of bitterness is related to the patient's feeling of dependence on the doctor for his own health and even his life.

This new critical attitude is reflected in the press, television, virtually all the mass media, and, increasingly, in government. The "money-grabbing" doctor and the one "who will not respond to a night house call" have become the standard butt of nightclub jokes. Government, especially Congress and the state legislatures, has been notably reluctant to antagonize or even criticize doctors in the past. It is now becoming more critical.[19] Moreover, patients and government alike are beginning to do something about their grievances. Controls on physicians' charges in publicly financed programs are gradually being introduced (Chapter 4). According to a *Medical World News* survey, complaints to local medical societies "rose 30 to 50 percent in the last three years."[20]

Many doctors, on their side, are increasingly critical of the "lay press" and "lay interference" in medicine. Many resent the patient whose illness is chronic and "uninteresting" or whose organic disease is complicated by emotional or socioeconomic problems. The reason is fairly simple. All the priorities—determined by traditional medical education, research money, physician interest, and even traditional patient demand—have always been given to the acute episode. As a result, while modern medicine can perform open-heart surgery and do 12 to 15 blood chemistries a minute, it cannot cure the common cold, overcome chronic constipation, or remedy some common foot disorders. Nor can it provide a quick cure for various neuroses. The patient with a chronic or emotional illness takes more time. He cannot be cured with a single prescription. In many cases, he cannot be cured at all, a frustrating experience for the doctor who measures his success in terms of numbers of patients cured, or at least the number seen.

To some doctors, perhaps the most disturbing aspect of the current situation is the ominous spread of malpractice suits—some 7,000 to 10,000 are now reported to be filed annually; the increasing generosity of juries—a Florida woman was recently awarded $1.5 million against two attending surgeons and a hospital on the grounds that she was paralyzed by an overdose of a drug following an operation;[21] and the dramatic nationwide rise in the cost of malpractice insurance. For doctors practicing in New York State a 65 percent rise went into effect September 1970, following a 55 percent increase in 1969. In California a 95 percent increase in 1968 was followed by a 110 percent rise in 1969.[22] In some jurisdictions it is reported that some doctors cannot get insurance at any price. Where this occurs, the underlying causes of the problem are further exacerbated: the inadequate pool of doctors is further depleted; the costs of care are further increased; and nothing is done to remedy either the actual malpractice or the breakdown in the doctor-patient relationship, which generally causes the suits in the first place.[23]

One limit on the doctor's productivity we have almost surely reached—the number of hours that he can be expected to work. Probably less of his current 63-hour week is spent on direct patient care than in the past and more on professional meetings, hospital staff work, and reading. However, this is all part of his continuing education and essential to the maintenance of high-quality care. It is not to the advantage of either doctor or patient to expect him to work longer hours.

The New Medical Humanism

Much publicity has been given recently to the "new medical student," the highly articulate, highly visible minority who belong to the Student Health Organization, the Medical Committee on Human Rights, and may even make up a majority of the Student American Medical Association. By a concern for family medicine and community medicine, for ghetto dwellers and poor people everywhere, for general problems of war and civil rights and social justice, and by an eagerness to try to do something about the physician's responsibility to society generally, this new breed of student and house staff has given hope to many critics of the profession that a fundamental change in professional orientation and ethical values may be in the making. Obviously, it is too soon to say. Other generations of idealistic medical students have turned into "realists" as life's pressures mounted. Nor do we know how large a proportion the present student activists represent of all students.

Fortunately, there are also other encouraging straws in the wind. For the first time in many years, "mainstream medicine" has developed its own self-critics—competent doctors, identified with organized medicine, but willing and able to speak out on the need for reforms. For example, Dr. John H. Knowles, General Director, Massachusetts General Hospital, one of the best known of this new type of medical leaders, said recently:

> No more than 20 percent of our physicians are completely attuned to the position of the AMA's board of trustees and AMPAC [American Medical Political Action Committee]. I think in the 70s the other physicians will make themselves heard, either by forcing a more sensitive response to their beliefs from the AMA or by choosing other methods and perhaps other organizations to make their views known.[24]

Both of these predictions appear to be materializing.

In a wonderfully funny put-on of the MD-entrepreneur, California GP Myron Greengold tells how he raised himself from a simple practitioner to the chief of an enterprise—himself, incorporated—listed on the Cow Counties Stock Exchange:

> How does it feel to be a 100 percent publicly owned OBG man? Well, I don't know how I ever practiced any other way. The rich bond between doctor and stockholder cannot be equaled in any other form of practice. When one of my owners gets a little cystocele or prolapse, she doesn't have to think twice about which doctor can do her the most good.[25]

This sort of humor was not often heard from the medical profession even a few years ago. An important element in the growing objectivity has to do with continued affluence. It should be noted as a significant phenomenon that the medical profession—the entire profession—has become the first in the nation to achieve a *de facto* guaranteed annual income. Obviously this was not a matter of conscious policy. Yet this is the net result of the many factors involved in the supply situation and the price of medical services. With all United States physicians—good, bad, and indifferent—now averaging on the order of $40,000 a year just from professional income, it is clear that motivations other than financial necessity are coming into play.

The MD-businessmen are concentrating on the stock market—or were, until the 1970 doldrums. The MD-politicians are manning various barricades—to the left as well as to the right. But for many good dedicated doctors, the relative freedom from financial strain, combined with the unrelenting physical strain, is calling for a reordering of personal priorities. Delving into the whys and wherefores of rising physician fees, one insightful management consultant writes:

> Many doctors are overgenerous to their families in order to compensate for the lack of time devoted to them. As this family time shrinks, there's greater pressure to earn and give still more and therefore greater upward pressure on fees.[26]

But more and more doctors, especially those with college-age, rebellious children, are now asking themselves if it wouldn't be better to cut down on the hours of work, and even earnings, in order to spend more time with their families. Others want to spend more time on community and similar unpaid activities. In short, it seems entirely possible that, with all doctors now virtually guaranteed a good living, they will stop worrying so much about fees, "third-party controls," the "corporate practice of medicine," the "unfair competition" of nurses and other health professionals, and all the other petty concerns that until very recently were the side effects of a long, harsh apprenticeship, a life of hard work, insufficient leisure, and a now thoroughly obsolete theory of scarcity economics.

In any case, the new humanism—both that of the student idealists (who, not so incidentally, have won for themselves the highest graduate stipends in medical history) and their affluent fathers—is greatly to be welcomed as a long-overdue reaction to over-preoccupation with Scientific Medicine and Entrepreneurial Medicine. However, if past history tells us anything, it is that idealism alone is not an adequate guarantor of social usefulness. To be effective, personal idealism must be translated into organizational policy and institutional structure.

*   *   *

Here, then, is Paradox Number One: More and better trained doctors than ever before, performing many near-miracles, seeing more patients, earning more money, and with a heartening infusion of new humanism; but a continuously increasing imbalance between supply and demand that is producing tremendous emotional and financial pressures, resentment on the part of both doctors and patients, and public depreciation of the medical profession: a dangerous situation that could easily turn the new idealism into frustrated cynicism.

NOTES

1. American Medical Association, Department of Survey Research, *Selected Characteristics of the Physician Population, 1963 and 1967* (Chicago: the Association, 1968), p. 10.

2. Haynes, M. A., Distribution of black physicians in the U.S., 1967. *J. Natl. Med. Assn.* Nov. 1969, p. 470.

3. *Med. Econ.,* Personal communication, Jan. 15, 1971. Figures are for all self-employed physicians under 65.

4. Public Health Service, U.S. Department of Health, Education, and Welfare, *Health Manpower U.S. 1965-67,* Pub. No. 1000, Series 14, No. 1, Nov. 1968, pp. 16-18. Data from AMA Department of Survey Research. Although precise figures for 1968 and 1969 are not yet available, preliminary analysis indicates that the proportion of physicians actually engaged in patient care has fallen more than was realized, as a result of more retirements and more full-time research.

5. *Amer. Med. News,* June 22, 1970, p. 8.

6. *Ibid.*

7. India and Singapore now prohibit the Educational Council for Foreign Medical Graduates from giving examinations in their countries, although many of their citizens contrive to take them elsewhere. No examinations may be given in the Arab countries at the present time.

8. *New York Times,* Feb. 11, 1969.

9. Public Health Service, U.S. Department of Health, Education, and Welfare, *Health Manpower: Perspective 1967,* pp. 9, 75. See comment at Note 4.

10. Stevens, R., Medical specialization, medical manpower, and public policy, *Health of the Nation* (University of Minnesota Health Sciences Center, Minneapolis, 1968), pp. 43-44. See also, Owens, A., General surgeons: too many in the wrong places. *Med. Econ.,* July 20, 1970.

11. Public Health Service, U.S. Department of Health, Education, and Welfare, *Health Resources Statistics: Health Manpower and Health Facilities, 1968,* Pub. No. 1509, 1968, pp. 123, 132.

12. *New York Times,* June 23, 1970.

13. *Med. Econ.,* Sept. 30, 1968, p. 88.

14. American Medical Association, *Survey of Medical Groups in the U.S., 1965,* Special Statistical Series (Chicago: the Association, 1968), p. 9. The definition of a "group" in this survey is "three or more full-time physicians formally organized to provide medical care consultation, diagnosis and/or treatment through the joint use of equipment and personnel, and with the income from medical practice distributed in accordance with methods previously determined by members of the group."

15. *Health Resources Statistics, op. cit.* (Note 11), p. 124.

16. *Med. Econ.,* Continuing Survey, 1968, unpublished data.

17. *Health Resources Statistics, op. cit.,* Appendix.

18. What is general practice really like today? *Med. World News,* May 19, 1967, p. 38.

19. See, for example, 91st Congress, 1st Session, *Medicare and Medicaid: Problems, Issues, and Alternatives,* Report of the Staff to the Committee on Finance, U.S. Senate, Feb. 9, 1970.

20. The doctor: how the patient sees him. *Med. World News,* Jan. 5, 1968, p. 42. For the view that dissatisfaction is increasing only moderately, see series of articles, How patients feel about doctors today. *Med. Econ.,* May 11 and June 8, 1970.

21. Although malpractice was not involved in a recent $2.3 million award to a 21-year-old college student injured in an auto accident, the implications for malpractice damages are inescapable. The huge award was based in large part on the cost of institutional medical care over a life expectancy of 52 years, including round-the-clock nurses who, it was testified, would probably cost $100,000 a year by 2022. *Med. Econ.,* July 6, 1970.

22. *New York Times,* July 12, 1970.

23. For discussion of the relation of malpractice suits to the doctor-patient relationship, see, Somers, H. M. and A. R., *Doctors, Patients, and Health Insurance* (Brookings Institution, 1961), pp. 472-74. Also, Bernzweig, E. P., Relationship of malpractice claims to the delivery of health services, *The Pharos,* July 1969, pp. 90-93.

24. Knowles, J., The physician in the decade ahead. *Hospitals, J.A.H.A.,* Jan. 1, 1970, p. 58.

25. I'm 100 percent publicly owned! *Med. Econ.,* Oct. 13, 1969, p. 216.

26. Owens, A., The facts behind the big fee trends. *Med. Econ.,* Jan. 19, 1970, p. 83.

Chapter 2

THE PATIENT

> Life remains the one illness that cannot be cured. By curing a sick person, the doctor, by this very fact, puts him in a position to contract other diseases later on.
>
> HENRI PÉQUIGNOT, M.D.
> *Scientific and Social Aspects of Modern Medicine* (1954)

> People just didn't use to be sick as much as they are today. They died when they got sick and didn't live sick.
>
> WILLIE JOHNSON
> *Negro sharecropper,*
> *Columbia, Mississippi* (1968)

A Demographic Profile

The average patient of the early 1970s is as different from his grandfather as the armamentarium of the modern physician is from his grandfather's little black bag. The demographic facts and trends that underlie the modern patient's health needs, attitudes, and demands are generally known. However, they are so basic to an understanding of the current health care crisis that they require constant emphasis. Here are some of the most important:

• The total population increased from 76 million in 1900 to 205 million as of April 1, 1970.[1] Between 1960 and 1970 the rise was 25 million, or 14 percent. In the past few years the rate of increase has been slowing down markedly. The 1.0 percent increase during 1968 represents the smallest annual increment since 1940. Census Bureau projections for the future have also been revised downward. Still the projected future rise is substantial. The range for 1975 is currently 215 to 228 million; for 1985, 242 to 275 million.[2]

• There was a rapid and substantial fall in the death rate for all age groups in the first half of the 20th century. Between 1900 and the mid-1960s nearly 23 years were added to the average length of life. By the mid-1960s the crude death rate had fallen to 9.4 per 1000 and life expectancy at birth was 70.2 years. Since then, however, there has been a marked leveling-off of improvement and, in some years, even a reversal. In 1968, for example, the death rate was up to 9.6 and life expectancy was down to 70.1 years.[3] The primary reasons for the change in mortality trends are: (1) the near-conquest of diseases of infectious origins, and (2) the recent upward trend in death rates from the major chronic diseases, including heart disease, cancer, and diabetes, and from accidents and other violence.[4]

[1]For this and succeeding notes in this chapter, see page 25.

15

• The over-65 population continues to grow in both absolute and relative terms. By January 1970 there were 19.6 million in this age group,[5] nearly 10 percent of the civilian population compared to only 4 percent in 1900. Census Bureau projections are for 25 million in this age group by 1985.

• Since 1957, the birth rate has resumed its long-run downward trend, reversing the upswing of the 1940s and early 1950s. The 1968 rate was 17.4 per 1000, considerably below the Depression rates. That year, for the first time since 1946, the number of births fell below the 3.5 million mark. There are some indications, however, that the decline may have come to a halt in the latter part of 1968.[6] In any case, the rapidly rising number of women in the 20 to 29 age bracket—products of the post-World War II "baby boom"—assures an increasing number of births, regardless of the rate. Even in 1968, children under 15 constituted 29 percent of the white population, 38 percent of nonwhites. The median age for all Negroes in 1968 was 21.2 years compared to 28.8 for whites.

• The shift of population from rural to urban residence continues, although in the past few years the great migrations of the post-World War II decades appear to have slowed down considerably. As of mid-1970, about 65 percent of the population lived in a metropolitan area. Well over half of these, 35 percent of the United States total, lived in a suburb. The social and political importance of the ever-growing suburbs is just now becoming apparent. In mid-1970 they became the largest sector of the population, exceeding for the first time both central cities and rural America.[7]

• The proportion of nonwhites in the population rose from 10.2 percent in 1940 to 12.4 percent in 1970.[8] The principal cause is their significantly higher birth rate. In 1970, there were approximately 23 million black Americans. Increasingly they are living in northern metropolitan areas. In 1940, 77 percent of all Negroes lived in the South. By 1966, only 55 percent remained there.

Although blacks and other minority groups remain at a substantial disadvantage in terms of incomes, housing, educational and job opportunities, the differentials are slowly but unmistakably narrowing. For example, the nonwhite/white ratio for median family income—51 percent in 1958—rose, by 1968, to 63 percent.[9] The Negro/white disparity varied, in 1968, from 54 percent in the South to 75 percent in the North Central states and 80 percent in the West.

• The proportion of women continues to rise with the ever-increasing differential between male and female longevity. Between 1920 and 1967, life expectancy for males increased 13.4 years; for females, 19.6. In 1920, there were 104 men for every 100 women in the U.S. In 1967, there were only 96. The excess of women in the over-65 age group is startling: 100 to 76.

• Educational levels continue to rise. In 1947, only 33 percent of persons 25 and over had completed high school; in 1968, the proportion was 53 percent. For those 25 to 29, the proportion was 73 percent. During these same years, the proportion with four or more years of college nearly doubled.

• Employment has remained generally high throughout the past two decades except for two or three relatively brief recessions. By late 1969 the unemployment rate was down to 3.5 percent of the civilian labor force. Starting early in 1970, however, the rate rose gradually to 5.5 percent in September. Due partly to Administration measures to combat the previous inflation, partly to the beginning of cutbacks in military production, the outlook as of October 1970 is uncertain.

Throughout the years of prosperity, the Negro unemployment rate was twice that of whites. It was also much higher for young people than for adults. For example, one-third of Negro teen-agers living in central cities were unemployed in 1968 compared to only one-eighth of the whites.[10] However, in the layoffs of 1970, it appears that whites have been hit harder than blacks, who have often been excluded from the unionized, well-paid defense industries.

• Family incomes continued to rise through 1969. In 1947, the median income of families was $3031. In 1969, it was $9433.[11] At the earlier date, 26 percent of families had incomes of less than $3000 (in constant 1968 dollars); only 10 percent, $10,000 or more.[12] In 1968, the proportions were 10 percent and 40 percent. In 1947, the median for nonwhite families was $2514. In 1968, it was $5540.

• As family income rose, so did that of the nation. As late as 1940, the gross national product was only $100 billion. In 1950, it was $285 billion; in 1960, $504; in 1969, $932. Unless the 1970 recession becomes considerably deeper than anticipated, GNP should be approaching an annual rate of $1000 billion (one trillion) by the end of 1970.

• The number of poor persons declined by more than one-third between 1959 and 1968.[13] According to the federal government's definition of poverty—below $3553 for a nonfarm family of four in 1968—13 percent of Americans were poor in that year compared with 22 percent in 1959. However, the number was still distressingly high—about 25 million. The number of poor whites dropped by 42 percent while the number of poor blacks declined by 27 percent. By 1969, the estimated number of poor was down to 24 million, or 12 percent of the total population.[14]

Although black families constitute only a little over one-fourth of all poor families, a disproportionate number of blacks are poor. In 1968 only 8 percent of white families were below the poverty line compared to 29 percent of Negro families. In 1967, 30 percent of central-city Negroes and 55 percent of Negroes living outside the metropolitan areas were poor. About half of the population in central-city poverty areas was nonwhite in 1968, up from 43 percent in 1960.[15] About half of all the poor are children.[16]

• Despite the long period of prosperity, nearly full employment, and effective social insurance programs providing old-age pensions, survivor, disability, unemployment, and workmen's compensation benefits, the welfare rolls and welfare payments have continued to rise throughout the past two decades. The most dramatic increase has been in the program of Aid to Families of

Dependent Children. In 1969, welfare recipients totaled more than 11 million; half were children in AFDC.[17]

The number of families headed by women rose during the past decade, especially among Negroes. One-half of Negro female heads of families are separated or divorced compared with one-third of white female heads.[18] At incomes below $3000 only a half of Negro families are headed by a male compared with three-fourths of white families. At this income level only one-fourth of Negro children live with both parents. At higher income levels, however, three-fourths of Negro families are headed by men and both parents are usually present.

Changing Health Needs and Demands

The health status of the American patient reflects the impact of these demographic and socioeconomic trends. In turn, it influences these trends for the future. The apparent reversal of the long-range improvement in life expectancy has been noted. Although the change is small, it appears to be significant, especially for men—both white and black—in their most productive middle years and especially when compared to the experience of other nations. According to a study by the National Advisory Commission on Health Manpower, based on data mostly from the late 1950s and early 1960s, 17 nations are reported to have longer life expectancy, at birth, for males, than the United States.[19] Our comparative position appears to have worsened rather than improved during the past two decades.[20]

Much has been made recently of our equally poor and deteriorating international showing with respect to infant mortality. In 1964, we were eighteenth in a list of countries compared by the United Nations. Our rate of 24.8 per 1000 live births is often compared to Sweden, the best, with 14.2.[21] Even if the comparison is confined to white babies in the United States, we still come off badly with a 1964 rate of 21.6. While there are undoubtedly some minor differences in statistical techniques in some of these countries, the comparability of the figures, especially for the Western European nations, has been studied by the National Center for Health Statistics and no statistical artifacts can account for the size of the differentials.

The long-standing discrepancy between the white and nonwhite infant death rate in the United States has also been widely noted and criticized. Following are some basic facts. During the 1950s the discrepancy increased. Between 1950 and 1960 the rate for white babies fell 14.6 percent; that for nonwhites, only 2.9 percent.[22] During the 1960s, however, the relationship was at least stabilized. From 1960 to 1966, the rates for both whites and nonwhites fell 10 percent. Between 1966 and 1967, the improvement for nonwhites was greater than for whites—7.5 percent and 4.4 percent, respectively.[23]

The discrepancy still remains, worse than it was in 1950. There was, in 1967, an 82 percent excess of nonwhite infant mortality over white. But the excess was less than it had been in 1960. Also, by 1968, the overall infant death rate was down to 21.7, almost one-third below that of a decade ago.

The mounting death rates from chronic disease and the irony of exceptionally high infant death rates in the urban ghettos, often next door to a leading medical center with first-rate clinical facilities, underscore the relationship of health conditions to environmental and socioeconomic problems and the impossibility of correcting health deficiencies solely through improved medical care. The same conclusion must be drawn from many other leading health problems—the alarming increase in venereal disease, alcoholism, drug addiction, automobile accidents, lung cancer, heart disease, and other conditions closely related to poor health habits and, of course, war and violence.

Dr. John Knowles complains:

> We are in a tremendous epidemic of gonorrhea. We have nosed out the French as the No. 1 nation in alcoholism. Over half of our 120,000 deaths a year from accidents are related to alcoholism. (Accidents themselves rate as the fourth leading cause of death, and the first among persons under 45.) Mental illness has become a major disease; in a given community, 20 percent of the population can be suffering from some form of it. One in 12 persons will require hospitalization for mental illness during his lifetime.[24]

Homicide is conspicuously on the rise in the United States. In 1969, the rate was over 7 per 100,000, about 60 percent above the low point registered in the late 1950s.[25] Deaths from the narcotics epidemic in New York City, already higher than ever before, are still rising, and no abatement is in sight. Narcotics, chiefly heroin, are now the leading killer in New York's 15-to-35 age group. About one-fourth of the 950 narcotics deaths in 1969 occurred among teen-agers and 53 percent among those under 25, about double the percentages of 10 years ago.[26]

In a recent sophisticated econometric study of the relationship of mortality to medical care and to environmental variables, Auster, Leveson, and Sarachek conclude that the environmental variables—especially income and education—are far more important determinants of death rates than medical care.[27] Other authorities feel that pollution is now such a serious problem in the United States that it overshadows all other factors as a threat to health.

In any case, the American patient, as he presents himself to his doctor or clinic, is a complex amalgam of genetic and environmental influences. His health problems are clearly not just physiological and are not susceptible to one-dimensional physiological "cures."

Despite this complexity, however, his needs, demands, and even his attitudes toward health and health care can be fairly well predicted, at least for the next decade or so. The population increase alone dictates a significant rise in need and demand—a rise that will continue for the foreseeable future. So does the change in the population profile. Older people, babies and young children, and women in their child-bearing years all have more-than-average health needs.

Despite the decline in the birthrate that characterized the decade of the 1960s, progress in control of infant mortality and the large number of young mothers in the population have resulted in an extraordinarily high proportion of young children with their special health needs. This is particularly true of low-income and minority groups, with their higher-than-average incidence of broken families. The belated but now substantial increase in birth-control information available to such families could be a significant factor in reducing future need in this area.

The health needs and attitudes of Negroes are probably no more complex than those of other population groups. According to the National Health Survey, "observed differences in health characteristics [between blacks and whites] were related more to socioeconomic factors of the two population groups than to color."[28] Most health problems of Negroes are almost certainly environmental in origin, associated primarily with poverty, the lesser stability of the black family, which traces back to slavery, and the recent mass migrations from Southern farms to Northern ghettos. The appalling living conditions prevalent in many of the ghettos account for some of the darkest blots on the nation's health record. We are paying the price for generations of neglect and discrimination and will continue to do so for years to come, despite the recent improvement in the Negro's socioeconomic status.

Greater moral and intellectual sensitivity to the problems of such groups, along with their increasing economic and political power, have dramatized the special and often overwhelming health needs of millions of the poor—not only blacks, but Spanish-Americans, Indians, and poor whites, especially in rural areas such as Appalachia.[29] Some 40 to 50 percent of the American people—the aged, children, the dependent poor, and those with some significant chronic disability—are in categories requiring relatively large amounts of medical care but with inadequate resources to purchase such care.

Meanwhile, the demands of the general population continue to grow. Industrialization and urbanization, rising incomes, better communications, and higher educational levels have all contributed to the "revolution of rising expectations" with respect to health services.

We are all familiar with the changing pattern of morbidity. The decline in acute contagious disease has been accompanied by a large relative increase in chronic illness. The Metropolitan Life Insurance Company puts it this way:[30]

> At the present time the chances at birth of a male eventually dying from a chronic disease are 83 in 100 in the United States, compared with 52 in 100 at the turn of the century. This probability has remained virtually unchanged during the past 20 years. The corresponding chances of dying from an acute condition are 6 in 100, which is about a sixth of such likelihood in 1901.

No one knows how many chronically ill there are. The National Health Survey reports that an estimated 96 million persons, nearly half the population, had one or more chronic diseases or impairments in 1966-67.[31]

Many of these people can and do lead nearly normal lives. But many others are more handicapped than they need be, probably die sooner than necessary, and surely lead more dependent, less useful lives than necessary, because of inadequate health care.

Despite the relative decline in infectious disease, acute illness and injury continue to afflict most Americans to a greater or lesser extent. In 1967 the incidence rate was 190 per 1000 persons.[32] As a result of chronic and acute illness combined, the average American had 15.3 days of restricted activity in 1967, including 5.7 days in bed.[33]

The Revolution of Rising Expectations

The continuing rise in the demand for health services, especially physicians' services, inherent in these basic demographic and health statistics, is further stimulated by two additional factors: our changed attitudes toward health and health care and greater financial support for health care.

The importance of greater financial support in creating the new patient cannot be overemphasized. People have always needed health services, but it is only in the past few decades, when health insurance, Medicare, Medicaid, and the numerous other public and private financing programs became available, that these needs have been generally translated into "effective demand." The growth of such effective demand since World War II has been very great, and there is a hen-and-egg mutually reinforcing relationship between this factor and the ever-rising expectations. There are few signs of any retrenchment in this respect (see Chapter 4).

Meanwhile, our standards and even our definition of health rise constantly. No longer are we content with the mere absence of serious disease. We want energy, vitality, even perpetual youth and beauty. At the same time, we have come, as a people, to believe that health care is a "right" rather than a "privilege." The more effective a service becomes, the more certain it is to be identified with "human rights."

Twenty-five years ago, there were those who took exception to the World Health Organization statement that "enjoyment of the highest attainable standard of health is one of the fundamental rights of every human being without distinction of race, religion, political belief, economic or social condition." Today virtually no one in public life would dare to question the American government's 1966 commitment, spelled out in P.L. 89-749, "to assure comprehensive health services of high quality for every person."

This obviously generates additional demand, some feel unreasonably so. Some economists and even doctors criticize what they call the "medicated survival" of our chronically ill and aged. True, many do live a purposeless, vegetative existence. But many others are highly productive despite serious physical infirmities. In our technological society brain is more important than brawn, and a polio victim can fill with distinction the highest office in the land.

In this day of organ transplants, cosmetic surgery, electronically controlled heart pacemakers and other remarkable and remarkably expensive mechanical appliances, designed to keep us alive, and hopefully productive, despite aging and chronic disabilities, we are unlikely to see any turning back in this revolution of rising expectations.

The New Hazards of Affluence

The influence of national prosperity, rising personal incomes and educational levels on health needs and use is complex and difficult to define. There is abundant documentation, from the National Center for Health Statistics and elsewhere, of the greater incidence of illness among the poor compared to those with higher incomes. According to Louis Harris, public opinion analyst, the incidence of serious illness is reportedly two to three times higher for the poor than for the population as a whole.[34]

The steady improvement in income and educational levels should, therefore, be expected to lead to lesser health needs per capita. Thus far, however, there has been no evidence of any such development. On the contrary, rising income levels have been associated with rising use patterns. In part, this is due to a catching up with a backlog of the long-neglected needs of those formerly denied access to needed services. In part, it is due to the higher standards of health and health care associated with higher incomes and educational levels. Moreover, at our present stage of development, affluence appears to produce its own threats to health—overeating, misuse of drugs (by the general population as well as teen-agers), underexercising, poor use of leisure, and so forth—no less than poverty does, perhaps more so.

The Auster-Leveson-Sarachek study (page 19) found that while more education is associated with relatively low death rates, high income is associated with high mortality when education and medical care are held constant, and concludes, "Adverse factors associated with the growth of income may be nullifying beneficial effects of increases in the quantity and quality of care."[35]

Dr. Michael Halberstam, writing in the *New York Times,* made the point even more graphically:

> Our mortality figures reflect convincingly the fact that most Americans die of excess rather than neglect or poverty.[36]

As part of his evidence he points to the comparative life expectancies for American men and women.

> Since distribution, financing, and quality of care is certainly equal for men and women in the U.S. . . . it is not medical care which accounts for the poor showing of American white men but rather "cultural patterns."

The American Heart Association recently reported that in a two-year study of 10,000 workers in the Chicago area, 30 percent were found to be "high risk candidates" for a heart attack. Three thousand of the workers suffered from two or more of the risk factors associated with heart attacks: cigarette smoking, high blood pressure, high cholesterol levels in the blood, overweight, diabetes, and abnormalities in the heart's electrical activity. Ten percent had three or more risk factors. This means, according to a formula based on the well-known Framingham (Mass.) heart survey, that these persons run a risk of heart attack that is ten times normal.[37]

Regardless of whether one accepts fully the growing threat of the "affluencia consumeritis syndrome," there appears no question but that continued prosperity will lead to significantly increased, rather than diminished, demand for health care.

The factors discussed in this chapter—demographic, economic, cultural, and political—have combined to create a virtual explosion of demand. This surge is reflected in the dramatic rise in utilization characteristic of the past several decades, applying to virtually all categories of health services and goods—physician visits, hospitalization, drugs, nursing homes, and so forth. Only in the past four or five years have we begun to see a possible leveling-off in the two major categories, physician visits and hospitalization.

The National Center for Health Statistics reports a slight decline in the number of patient visits per capita between fiscal year (FY) 1964 and FY 1967. The average for the later date was 4.3 per year compared to 4.5 three years earlier.[38] There was a similar development in the rate of hospital admissions (see Chapter 3). This possibly important change in use patterns has been largely obscured by the continual price rises in both categories and the resulting dramatic increase in national and family expenditures (see Chapter 4). It merits careful study.

In any case, the result of the long-run trend toward greater use has not always been improved health. The discrepancy between rate of expenditure for health and improvement in health status appears to be increasing. Part of the problem relates to our still unassimilated affluence. Part of it relates to the also unassimilated mass migrations. Part has to do with the continuing irrationality and irresponsibility of many consumers who find it easier to rely on the age-old "bottle-of-medicine fetish" than practice the self-control essential to good health.

The Alienated Consumer-Patient

> Wherever people live, the rising expectations of which we hear so much have risen particularly steeply with regard to health. Of all the issues that confront Americans, this one cuts most widely across racial, political, age and income lines in every section of the country. And of all the gaps between promise and performance, this is the one that the vital center of the nation—whether because care is unavailable or impersonal and expensive—finds most deeply disappointing.
>
> JUDITH RANDALL
> *Syndicated newspaper column* (July 16, 1970)

A considerable part of the problem, as well as part of the reason for the persistent consumer irrationality, is the fact that so many people still lack access to good health care. For many it is quantitatively deficient. For many more, including many in middle-income and upper-income categories, it is qualitatively lacking, particularly in the educational influence of a good doctor-patient relationship, a lack that probably disturbs the patient even more than it does the doctor.

In view of the widespread belief among health professionals as well as among affluent Americans generally that the poor are irresponsible in health affairs, two of the findings from the Harris health survey are significant:[39]

1. The poor actually place a higher priority on trying to achieve a healthy status than others.

> Ironically, the only group to give good health as precious a place in the order of life values as the poor are those at the opposite end of the spectrum, the affluent with incomes over $10,000 who have had some college education. For example, 59 percent of the poor blacks and 72 percent of poor whites give health a higher priority than having a good job, compared with 51 percent of the American people as a whole.

2. Most of the poor have confidence in modern medicine and the modern doctor. But they feel excluded. Seventy-four percent of the poor feel that "most doctors don't want you to bother them." Over and over, from Harlem to Appalachia to the Spanish-American enclaves of the Southwest, there is the same refrain, "Not enough doctors! Impersonal clinics! Professional indifference! Waiting . . . waiting . . . waiting! You could die before they get to you!"

Similar findings were reported by the Division of Regional Medical Programs on the basis of student surveys in a number of poverty communities during the summer of 1968. For example:

> The community residents (both urban and rural) seemed surprisingly sophisticated (i.e., above students' expectations) about the use of health services. This was particularly true of urban mothers using hospital clinics for their children. It might be described as "utilization savvy."
>
> All projects found an overwhelming perceived need for ambulatory care services that were convenient, competent, and courteous. . . . Patients will travel farther (passing two other hospitals) to go to a third hospital outpatient department which they feel "accepts" them.
>
> The community is less interested in the content of care (the chlorine level of the swimming pool or the use of specific antibiotics) than in the setting of that care (accessibility, appropriateness, and affability).
>
> Most of the communities felt they were oversurveyed and underserviced.[40]

Not surprisingly, many a patient, especially if he is one of the millions with a chronic disability, feels abandoned,[41] frustrated, fatalistic about health problems, often angry at the providers; and so, as already noted in Chapter 1, the number of malpractice suits rises. Even those patients who win their suits receive very limited benefits. According to one federal study, only about 30 percent of the money paid out by insurance companies in malpractice awards goes to the patient; the rest goes to the lawyers.[42] In any case, the net effect on the general quality of care is probably close to zero while the net effect on costs is substantial.

Through unions, employee benefit plans, neighborhood health centers, welfare organizations, and others, consumers have been groping for some way to make their grievances heard and to obtain a greater degree of responsible representation in medical care institutions. Some progress has been made. "Patient power," according to some, is already making itself felt—even at AMA meetings! As this is written, portions of New York City's Lincoln Hospital are being "occupied" by a group of militant young Puerto Ricans whose motivations include fully justified demands for improvements in the health services available in their community along with a play for power and publicity.

The Joint Commission on Accreditation of Hospitals has set up an advisory board made up of people who use hospital services—"a revolutionary idea for the 51-year-old organization that previously had considered that its only obligation was to hospitals and the medical profession."[43] Mark Berke, President of the American Hospital Association, has recommended that the Association set up a "council on consumer interests, coequal with all other councils in our structure."[44]

Whether such developments, encouraging as they are, will lead to greater mutual understanding and a common attack on the nation's health care problems or will pass into history as only a temporary political expediency remains to be seen. In any case, a vast gulf in communication remains, especially between the poor and the medical care Establishment. The blame is not all on one side, but the fact remains that the traditional patterns of professional-consumer relations have not yielded substantially to the changing circumstances, and medical care remains almost entirely controlled by the providers. Even when government intervenes, ostensibly in the name of the consumer-patient, the intervention has not generally been very effective.

*   *   *

What all this adds up to is Paradox Number Two: A longer-lived, less disease-ridden, better educated, richer patient than ever before but, at the same time, needing and demanding more health care than ever before (this applies both to the affluent majority and the poor minority), increasingly critical of existing health care institutions, and determined to change these institutions, by whatever means he can command, in order to get what he thinks he needs.

NOTES

1. U.S. Department of Commerce, Bureau of the Census, *Population Estimates and Projections*, Series P-25, No. 445, May 20, 1970, p. 1.

2. U.S. Department of Commerce, Bureau of the Census, *Statistical Abstract of the U.S., 1969*, p. 8. Unless otherwise indicated, statistical data in Chapter 2 are from this source.

3. Metropolitan Life Insurance Co., *Stat. Bull.*, Mar. 1969, p. 7.

4. See, U.S. Department of Health, Education, and Welfare, National Center for Health Statistics, *The Change in Mortality Trend in the U.S.*, USPHS Pub. 1000, Series 3, No. 1, 1964. Also, *Mortality Trends in the U.S., 1954-63*, Pub. 1000, Series 20, No. 2, 1966.

5. U.S. Department of Health, Education, and Welfare, *Soc. Secur. Bull.*, Apr. 1970, p. 74.

6. Metropolitan Life Insurance Co., *Stat. Bull.*, Feb. 1969, p. 5.

7. *New York Times*, June 21, 1970.

8. Bureau of the Census, *Population Estimates and Projections*, Series P-25, No. 442, Mar. 20, 1970, p. 11.

9. U.S. Department of Commerce and U.S. Department of Labor, *The Social and Economic Status of Negroes in the U.S., 1969*, BLS No. 375, and Bureau of the Census, *Current Population Reports*, Series P-23, No. 29, 1970, p. 14.

10. Bureau of the Census, *Special Studies*, Series P-23, No. 27, Feb. 7, 1969, p. v.

11. Bureau of the Census, *Consumer Income*, Series P-60, No. 70, July 16, 1970, p. 3.

12. Bureau of the Census, *Consumer Income*, Series P-60, No. 66, Dec. 23, 1969, p. 20.

13. Bureau of the Census, *Consumer Income*, Series P-60, No. 68, Dec. 31, 1969, p. 1 ff.

14. Bureau of the Census, *Current Population Reports*, Series P-20, No. 204, July 13, 1970, p. 1.

15. *Special Studies, op. cit.*, p. vi.

16. Orshansky, M., The poverty roster. *Sources: A Blue Cross Report on Health Problems of the Poor* (Chicago: Blue Cross Association, 1968), p. 4. See this whole publication for an imaginative report.

17. U.S. Department of Health, Education, and Welfare, *Soc. Secur. Bull.*, June 1970, p. 41.

18. *The Social and Economic Status of Negroes in the U.S., 1969, op. cit.*, p. 71 ff.

19. National Advisory Commission on Health Manpower, *Report*, Vol. I, pp. 91-92. According to this source, the number of countries with longer life expectancy for males than the United States is given as 20. I have excluded two—Israel and New Zealand—since, in these nations, not all residents are counted in the statistics. Also, Puerto Rico is illogically listed as a separate nation.

20. Rutstein, D., *The Coming Revolution in Medicine* (Cambridge: MIT Press, 1967), pp. 15-28.

21. U.S. Department of Health, Education, and Welfare, National Center for Health Statistics, *International Comparison of Perinatal and Infant Mortality: The U.S. and Six West European Countries*, Pub. No. 1000, Series 3, No. 6, Mar. 1967, p. 2.

22. Bureau of the Census, *Statistical Abstract of the U.S., 1968*, p. 55.

23. Bureau of the Census, *Statistical Abstract of the U.S., 1969*, p. 55.

24. *Look*, June 2, 1970, p. 74.

25. Metropolitan Life Insurance Co., *Stat. Bull.*, Mar. 1970, p. 7.

26. *New York Times,* June 21, 1970.

27. Auster, R., Leveson, I., and Sarachek, D., The production of health, an exploratory study. *J. Human Resources,* Fall 1969, p. 430.

28. U.S. Department of Health, Education, and Welfare, National Center for Health Statistics, *Differentials in Health Characteristics by Color, U.S., 1965-67,* USPHS Pub. No. 1000, Series 10, No. 56, 1969, p. 1.

29. See, Leo, P. A. and Rosen, G., A bookshelf on poverty and health. *Amer. J. Public Health,* Apr. 1969, p. 591.

30. Metropolitan Life Insurance Co., *Stat. Bull.,* May 1969, p. 4.

31. U.S. Department of Health, Education, and Welfare, National Center for Health Statistics, *Current Estimates from the Health Interview Survey, U.S., July 1966-June 1967,* USPHS Pub. No. 1000, Series 10, No. 43, p. 3.

32. *Ibid.,* p. 2.

33. *Ibid.,* pp. 3-4.

34. Harris, L., Living sick. *Sources: A Blue Cross Report on Health Problems of the Poor, op. cit.,* (Note 16), p. 24.

35. Auster *et al., op. cit.,* pp. 411-12.

36. Halberstam, M., The MD should not try to cure society. *New York Times Mag.,* Nov. 9, 1969, p. 62 ff.

37. *New York Times,* Mar. 22, 1970.

38. U.S. Department of Health, Education, and Welfare, *Volume of Physician Visits, U.S., July 1966-June 1967,* USPHS Pub. 1000, Series 10, No. 49, p. 1.

39. Harris, *op. cit.,* pp. 22, 30.

40. U.S. Department of Health, Education, and Welfare, Division of Regional Medical Programs, *News Information Data,* Oct. 24, 1969, pp. 3-5.

41. For discussion of four categories of patients who feel particularly "abandoned," see Somers, A. R., The missing ingredient. *Med. Opinion and Review,* Aug. 1969, p. 27.

42. *New York Times,* July 12, 1970.

43. *The Washington Post,* June 18, 1970.

44. Incoming President Mark Berke's inaugural address, *Hospitals, J.A.H.A.,* Mar. 16, 1970, p. 63.

Chapter 3

THE HOSPITAL

The impact on patterns of medical care in America wrought by the hospital . . . probably exceeds that of all . . . other social entities. Certainly the average physician and the way he does his work have been more widely influenced by hospitals than by any other form of social organization. The force of the hospital is felt not only on the doctor's management of his own private patients who are hospitalized, but on the whole fabric of health service organization in the community.

MILTON I. ROEMER, M.D.
Hospital Progress (September 1964)

Although it comes from an ancient tradition, the modern hospital, in fully recognizable form, is less than fifty years old.

At most it will last, in fully recognizable form, another decade or so. But by then, almost surely, what is different from the present will overshadow what is similar. And we may expect these changes to represent more than improved technology and differently trained personnel. For there will certainly be a change in the function of hospitals, just as there has been a change in function during the past half century.

MICHAEL CRICHTON, M.D.
Five Patients: The Hospital Explained (1970)

Of all present developments in the health care field, the emergence of the modern hospital has been the most dramatic and the most impressive example of the institutionalization of medical care. Within living memory an age-old institution for the custodial care of the sick poor has emerged as the center of the medical world—a vast complex of expensive buildings, specialized equipment, and interdisciplinary skills brought together for inpatient and outpatient care, research, professional and general health education.

Professional Center of the Health Care World

The doctor's indispensable workshop, the hospital is also the principal center for development of quality measurements and controls. Its complex of internal and external audits and standards constitutes the nation's primary protection against unqualified or inappropriate medical practice.

The reality of this situation was explicitly affirmed by the Supreme Court of Illinois in 1965 in the historic Darling case in the following words:

"The conception that the hospital does not undertake to treat the patient, does not undertake to act through its doctors and nurses, but undertakes instead simply to procure them to act upon their own responsibility, no longer reflects the fact.

27

Present-day hospitals, as their manner of operation plainly demonstrates, do far more than furnish facilities for treatment. They regularly employ on a salary basis a large staff of physicians, nurses and interns, as well as administrative and manual workers, and they charge patients for medical care and treatment, collecting for such services, if necessary, by legal action. Certainly, the person who avails himself of hospital facilities expects that the hospital will attempt to cure him, not that its nurses or other employees will act on their own responsibility." The Standards for Hospital Accreditation, the state licensing regulations and the defendant's bylaws demonstrate that the medical profession and other responsible authorities regard it as both desirable and feasible that a hospital assume certain responsibilities for the care of the patient.[1]

The Illinois Court was not the first to enunciate this doctrine. A New York court had done so as early as 1957[2] and a California court in 1958.[3] The first part of the passage just cited was quoted by the Illinois Court from the New York decision. The earlier cases did not attract widespread attention, probably because they were about a decade ahead of public opinion. But the Darling case has been widely hailed as marking legal recognition of a *de facto* situation. The modern hospital, in more and more jurisdictions, is held legally and financially responsible for the quality of care rendered by all employed or affiliated health personnel, including physicians.[4]

The Rise and Leveling-Off of Inpatient Use

The public's appreciation of this new role of the hospital is reflected in the utilization statistics, for both inpatient and outpatient care. Between 1931 and 1962, the annual rate of inpatient admissions to general hospitals (all except mental and tuberculosis) went up steadily from 56 per 1000 population to 140 per 1000, or 150 percent.[5] Thanks to a decline in the average length of stay, however, from 15.3 days to 9.3, the total number of patient days per year per 1000 population rose at a much slower pace, from 860 to 1295, or approximately 51 percent.

In recent years, Medicare, Blue Cross, and other third-party payers have tried to restrain the rise in inpatient use through various forms of utilization control. Utilization review procedures are now required for accreditation by the Joint Commission on Accreditation of Hospitals and for participation in Medicare.

The American Hospital Association and the hospital industry have generally cooperated, especially through promotion of voluntary hospital planning to hold down construction of new hospital beds. As a result of these efforts, inpatient utilization rates have increased much more slowly in recent years. The admission rate for community hospitals rose only 25 percent from 1947 to 1967.[6] The ratio has been virtually stationary, at about 138 per 1000, since 1964. However, the average length of stay for community hospitals, after dropping to 7.6 days, 1958-62, increased again to 8.4 in 1968.[7]

There is also a striking and persistent regional variation in hospital use. In some states, the population receives twice as many days of general hospital care as in other states. For example, in 1966, the number of days of care per 1000 population in Delaware was 1984; in Rhode Island, 1947; and in Massachusetts, 1655.[8]

[1]For this and succeeding notes in this chapter, see page 37.

By contrast, the figure for New Mexico was 768; for Idaho, 830; and for Utah and Mississippi, 823. The contrast does not involve any significant variation in admission rates. It arises almost entirely from the difference in average length of stay. For example, the National Center for Health Statistics reports a national average, for 1965, of 7.8, a high of 9.1 in the Northeast, and a low of 6.8 in the West.[9] Factors that may enter into this significant differential include the extent to which care for the chronically ill is alternatively given in hospitals or nursing homes, differences in the age composition of the population, degree of urbanization, differences in per capita income, and differences in the number of doctors and hospital beds.

The Dramatic Growth of Outpatient Services

By comparison with the leveling-off of inpatient use, outpatient visits have continued to skyrocket. During the same period, 1947-67, the rate per 1000 rose from 223 to 562, six times as fast as the rise in inpatient admissions. In 1953, there were two outpatient visits for every inpatient admission; by 1967, the ratio had increased to four to one.[10] In 1953, only about 60 percent of all community hospitals reported outpatient services; by 1967, the number had increased to 90 percent. These developments are particularly significant in view of the many professional and financial obstacles—such as inadequate insurance coverage—to the expansion of hospital ambulatory services.

Hospital ambulatory services have traditionally been classified in three categories: those provided in organized outpatient clinics, in emergency rooms, and special diagnostic and treatment services, including laboratory, x-ray, and physical therapy, provided to private patients on a referral basis. Used for the most part by the indigent, the outpatient departments (OPDs) have long been a principal site of medical education. Although once considered an adequate source of care for the poor, they have, in recent years, come under increasing criticism from both patients and physicians. In absolute numbers, clinic visits have continued to increase over the past decade. As a proportion of total outpatient visits in community hospitals, however, they fell from 48 percent in 1957 to 39 percent in 1968.[11]

The hostility and bitterness often expressed toward these clinics, especially by the poor, is probably more a reflection of rising consumer purchasing power and expectations and higher community standards than any actual decline in quality. Whatever the reasons, however, the traditional OPD clinic is now generally considered obsolete and many hospitals, including most of the prestigious teaching institutions, are groping for acceptable substitutes.

The two other types of hospital ambulatory services have demonstrated vigorous growth. Neither was indigent-oriented. Emergency room visits in community hospitals rose about 148 percent between 1957 and 1968. As a proportion of all reported outpatient visits, they rose from 21 percent to 34 percent.

This is highly revealing as to public demand, because this is the one type of hospital service that the public can get without the assistance of professional "gatekeepers" who guard the doors against "improper" use of all other hospital services. The bulk of the increase does not reflect any significant rise in major trauma or accidents in our society. From a purely medical point of view, most of this demand does not represent emergencies at all. It is for the type of physician service typically associated with private office practice. In part it reflects a demand for instant care at the convenience of both physician and patient. From the doctor's point of view, the OPD permits him to see patients on weekends and other times when his office is not scheduled to be open. Equally important, or perhaps even more so, many doctors feel they can do a better job in the emergency room if there is anything seriously, or potentially seriously, wrong with the patient. It also reflects the frequent lack of availability of doctors when needed and the lack of insurance coverage for other types of ambulatory care.

There are no comparable national statistics to show the rise in ambulatory services provided on a referral basis by the various diagnostic and treatment departments. Indeed, many hospitals do not distinguish in their records between inpatient and outpatient services of this type and therefore have not noted the extent of this change in demand. It has been going on, however, in almost all the specialized departments. The x-ray department has been most dramatically affected. A 1967 survey of all Philadelphia hospitals indicates that 49 percent of all diagnostic x-ray procedures were performed for outpatients. For Philadelphia General Hospital, the percentage was 62.[12]

Ambulatory patients are also referred to the hospital for laboratory tests, blood transfusions, oxygen therapy, physical and occupational therapy, social service consultations, dietary consultations, EKGs, minor surgery, even anesthesia in the form of nerve blocks, and so forth. Not all of this reflects qualitative improvement. Part of the increase in laboratory work, for example, may be related to its profitability. In general, however, it does indicate significant improvement in the quality of ambulatory care and, by the same token, the private physician's growing dependence on the hospital to help him carry on his regular practice. It is doubtful, however, that many hospitals are now equipped, in facilities, staff, or even in purpose, to meet this demand. Most specialist departments are still organized primarily for inpatient care. Too often, the individual seeking ambulatory care feels like a poor relative buying a suit of clothes in a large wholesale department, unwanted, a nuisance who represents an interruption in the routine.

In their totality, the outpatient services of the modern hospital now constitute one of its principal components, needed and demanded by both patients and physicians, an indispensable aspect of community health services, but still inadequately recognized in the hospital's organizational, financial, and prestige hierarchies and grossly downgraded in most health insurance programs.

De Facto Center of Community Health Services and Planning

Over and above all the services rendered on its own premises, the hospital now frequently finds itself involved in a growing network of community health programs and regional or areawide planning programs. Some of the better hospitals now provide or supervise home care programs, nursing homes, extended care facilities, mental health clinics, neighborhood health centers, and other special facilities for the poor.[13] The American Hospital Association has set up a special Committee on

Health Care for the Disadvantaged, paralleling the AMA's Committee on Health Care of the Poor.

For two decades, the AHA has been in the forefront of the hospital planning movement.[14] Most recently, it has sought to strengthen the planning process through its own proposal to tie planning to third-party reimbursement,[15] and through support of the Secretary's Advisory Committee on Hospital Effectiveness (Barr Committee) and its recommendations for tying voluntary areawide planning to state licensing authority and strengthening both through the use of federal funds.[16] Needless to say, not all AHA constituent bodies or member hospitals have been equally enthusiastic, especially when their own interests have been affected. By and large, however, it can be said that the great majority of the nation's hospitals are now committed, at least in principle, to health care planning at all levels.

The results, thus far, have not been impressive in terms of adequate and well-balanced community health services. Unnecessary duplication of expensive equipment, such as that necessary for open-heart surgery, persists alongside obvious gaps in facilities for primary care. But the hospitals' success in restraining new construction, especially of inpatient beds, in holding down inpatient admissions, and in raising occupancy rates,[17] testifies to their effectiveness in areas where policy has been fairly clear and a course of action defined.

A different approach to systemization is represented by the slow but unmistakable trend toward greater coordination among individual hospital units. This trend includes such varying degrees of consolidation as outright physical merger, satellite systems, hospital chains, affiliation agreements, and varying forms of contractual relations.[18] While consolidations of this sort, especially mergers, have proceeded much less rapidly than many hospital planners and economists would like to see, the pace has been stepped up during the 1960s.

The modern hospital is gradually, albeit somewhat reluctantly, becoming a community health center, whether as a part of a multi-institutional unit or a single autonomous institution. It is the one institution with the potential for providing or assuming responsibility for the provision of the full range of comprehensive health services—prevention, treatment, rehabilitation, and aftercare.

Rising Costs and Prices

Reflecting this enlarged role, the hospital is now the major consumer of the nation's health care dollar. In 1950, hospital operating expenses accounted for 30 percent of the dollar. By 1968, this had increased to 36 percent.[19] Construction costs added nearly 4 percent more. By 1969, well over 40 percent of all United States health care expenditures, at least $25 billion, were going into construction and maintenance of the nation's hospitals.

Ironically, but not surprisingly, the hospital's increasingly dominant role in health affairs and its increasing importance in the total United States economy have made it the target for a great deal of criticism as well as praise. The one aspect of hospital operations that has received the most unfavorable attention in recent years is the astronomical rise in costs. The average expense per *adjusted* patient day in community hospitals throughout the country rose 38 percent in only three years,

1965 to 1968. In 1968, the average was $55.80.[20] By February 1970, it reached $75.00.[21]

Needless to say, this rise in operating costs has been translated into patient costs or charges. In March 1970, the average daily service charge (room rate) was 279 percent higher than it was about 10 years earlier.[22] In 1965, according to a *New York Times* report, it cost New York City an average of $58.35 a day for each indigent bed patient. In 1969, the average was $97.00.[23] The care of a patient in the intensive care unit (ICU) at Strong Memorial Hospital, Rochester, N.Y., is reported to cost the hospital, although not the patient, some $300 a day, about three times the per diem average for the hospital as a whole.[24]

The full explanation of the rise in hospital costs—a mixture of greater complexity (for example, most patients in the Strong Memorial ICU are recovering from open-heart surgery, serious burns, or accidents with multiple trauma), higher quality, persistent inefficiency, and inflation—has never been adequately analyzed. It reflects such specific factors as rising labor costs; the increasing employment of more highly skilled personnel, including physicians; the changing status and higher pay of the house staff; the rise in the cost of construction, including the cost of borrowing money, and supplies of all types; the increasing use of computers and other expensive equipment; the increase in number and sophistication of diagnostic tests and therapeutic procedures; the changing mix of the patient population with a marked trend toward more serious illness; the increasing involvement of the community hospital in research, education, and community health services and planning; the shorter length of stay (although, as noted, this trend has now been reversed); the persistence of too many economically inefficient small units;[25] and the rising costs of administrative overhead, including such relatively new areas as public relations, personnel, and malpractice insurance.

Above all, there is the typically diffuse managerial structure which in turn derives from the tradition of dual control between the medical and administrative lines of authority, and which generally prevents the institution from fully employing the managerial controls essential to balance the new technologies and higher personnel earnings with increased productivity. On the contrary, the increased capital investment in hospitals in recent years has been accompanied by a steady rise in the personnel/patient ratio. Between 1963 and 1968, for example, the number of employees in community hospitals increased from 6.0 per 1000 adjusted patient days to 6.8, or by 13 percent.[26] The increase was all in the area of inpatient services.

A single example illustrates both the complexity of the cost problem and the difficulty of controlling it. Dr. John Romano has emphasized the growing complexity of hospital medical practice by contrasting the hospital records of two patients with similar diseases, one admitted in 1908, the other to the same hospital in 1938:

> The record of the first patient occupied two and one-half pages and comprised observations made by two clinicians (the attending and the house officer) and a pathologist-bacteriologist. The record of the second patient consisted of 29 pages, the observations of the visiting physicians, 5 house officers, 10 specialists, and 14 technicians, a total of 32 individuals.[27]

This was in 1938! By 1969, the record of such a patient often approaches the size of a large-city telephone book. The problems of automation, storage, retrieval, and general usefulness as well as the cost of the medical record have become formidable.

Statistical shortcomings, especially in the traditional index of changing costs, the average per diem, now discarded by the AHA, have probably overstated the cost increase. Whatever the explanations and extenuating circumstances, however, the rise has been real and substantial, as every third-party payer knows. The July 1970 settlement between the League of Voluntary Hospitals and Homes of New York and Local 1199 of the Drug and Hospital Union, providing increases of 25 to 30 percent over the next two years, is a portent of the future, unless new control factors are forthcoming.

Speculation as to the future varies from the conservative, a Social Security Administration estimate of a rise of only 70 percent by 1975,[28] to the not-so-tongue-in-cheek estimate by AHA President Mark Berke and former Assistant Secretary of HEW for Health and Scientific Affairs Philip Lee that, by 1980, costs would average $1000 a day in major urban hospitals, $600 in medium-sized communities, and $400 in rural areas.[29] There is, clearly, a widespread feeling that costs are now out of control and nobody knows what to do about it.

The recent rapid growth of for-profit hospital and nursing home chains in many parts of the country—there are now more than 100 such corporations engaged in the business of providing institutional health services[30]—has been hailed in some quarters as one answer to the cost problem through the injection of the profit motive, more unified management, and aggressive competition. Indeed, some of these new chains and individual hospitals have demonstrated an ability to operate at significantly lower costs than the nonprofit institutions. The latter claim, however, that this differential is due less to managerial efficiency than to a policy of patient selection which favors the less serious cases and avoids the aged and the indigent. While there is undoubtedly much to be said for the claims of the new corporations, neither they nor anyone else believes that the United States hospital system could be run exclusively, or even primarily, on a for-profit basis.

Growing Criticism of Hospitals

The impact of rising hospital costs on Blue Cross and other health insurance rates, their contribution to the alarming rise in the costs of Medicare and the difficulties and cutbacks in Medicaid, combined with growing criticism of the alleged depersonalization of care, have led to a veritable avalanche of public attacks on hospitals. Typical is the introduction to a *New York Times* article:

> A girl with a series of defects was taken to Jacobi Municipal Hospital 44 times during her first nine months of life and was never treated by the same physician twice. . . .

> "You come to this hospital and we're telling you somebody's going to take care of you," said Dr. Seymour M. Glick, Chief of Medicine at Coney Island Hospital, "The fact is, you're going to lie in a damp bed, develop an ulcer, septicemia [blood poisoning] and perhaps ultimately die because of inadequate nursing care."[31]

The targets here are municipal institutions, run primarily for the poor and particularly vulnerable both to bureaucratic inefficiency and to political attack. But criticism of the nongovernmental institutions is only a little less sensational. The most scholarly attack of the recent past was directed at one of the nation's leading teaching hospitals.[32] In fact, criticism of hospitals seems to have become almost a national obsession.

The waiting list for a medical or surgical bed in some hospitals and the empty bassinet or pediatric crib in others, the long hard bench in the OPD and the cost of an emergency room visit, the moonlighting resident, the invisible pathologist, the attending surgeon with privileges in several hospitals but primary loyalty to none, the newly militant nurse, the traditionally underpaid ward maid who is not so underpaid anymore but is still stuck in a dead-end job, the sometimes unnecessary cobalt unit, the necessary but still generally missing family health service: all of these and dozens of other issues, not always accurately, but dramatically, reported in the mass media, have now become arguments in the crescendo of public debate.

The hostility has been particularly bitter on the part of some of the poor, whose long-standing resentment against the indignities and impersonality of traditional outpatient care, as well as the low wages and poor working conditions traditionally associated with nonprofessional hospital labor, was suddenly released as the Office of Economic Opportunity and other new programs provided such groups with an opportunity for public expression for the first time.

Not all hospital critics are poor, however. During the past few years there has developed a more sophisticated body of opinion that downgrades the role of the hospital, partly because of the high costs, partly because it is still identified primarily with curative rather than preventive medicine, partly because it is alleged that the hospital has been unresponsive both to the health needs of the poor and to their need to participate at the decision-making level in basic community institutions, such as the hospital. The OEO neighborhood health center program with its emphasis on free-standing, community-controlled centers, entirely separate from the hospital, and the Comprehensive Health Planning Program (P.L.89-749), with its emphasis on "comprehensive" as opposed to personal health services and on community as opposed to provider control, embodied this point of view, especially in their early days.

Here are three examples of this high-level criticism:

> The hospital has outlived its usefulness and must be replaced by some other form of medical service. The hospital is now the focus of patient care but is obviously inadequate since costs are skyrocketing beyond any tolerance. Patients are admitted to the hospital today only because there is no alternative source of needed services.[33]

> I am seriously suggesting that the hospital as we now know it is an obsolete and ineffective institution for ambulatory care, and that hospitals for the future should be vastly different—in effect, intensive care units for patients with critical and complex illness. . . . The hub of the medical care universe would be a network of comprehensive community health centers.[34]

> We shall have to devise and put into practice new systems of organizing health services, including the facilities and institutions that provide them. Heretofore, the hospital—the great citadel of cure—has been considered the heart of the system. But if we envision a system which emphasizes health protection and advancement, admission to the hospital will be an admission of failure. The hospital will be the place of the last resort—essential but no longer dominant.[35]

Unfortunately for the therapeutic value of most of the criticism, it tends to be highly inconsistent and often contradictory. The hospital is accused, at one and the same time, of being "inefficient" and inadequately concerned with cost controls, and of being "heartless" and inadequately concerned with humane values. The large body of existing public regulation reflects this confusion and in many cases hurts rather than helps the situation.[36] Moreover, many of those who proclaim the need for integration of the community's health services into a unified comprehensive system while denying the role of leadership to the natural center of such a system —the hospital—offer no alternative or the alternative of a committee!

Ironically, this critical view of the hospital is also shared by many physicians who view the institution as "the enemy," and, according to some, even more to be feared than government. The opposition of the AMA to the appointment of Dr. John H. Knowles, General Director, Massachusetts General Hospital, to the office of Assistant Secretary of HEW for Health and Scientific Affairs, was a dramatic illustration of this attitude. It is evident in many examples of medical society opposition to the growing hospital responsibility. For example, some leaders of organized medicine insist that utilization and other peer review should be done not by hospital-medical staff committees but by committees of state or local medical societies. The AMA also opposes the AHA proposal to tie hospital reimbursement to areawide planning—one way to put some teeth into voluntary planning.[37]

Like most critics, however, the medical profession is ambivalent about the hospital. Alongside those doctors who would like to weaken the institution there are those, probably a much larger proportion, who recognize its inevitable role and, rather than trying to weaken it, seek to control it. The battle for control of the hospital, whether it is to be primarily a physicians' workshop or a community health center, has been going on for some years but grows sharper as the issues become clearer and the stakes larger. The recent rewriting of the Joint Commission on Accreditation of Hospitals Standards provided a new chapter in this old feud.

> The issue is joined on the question of whether medical staff representation on governing boards shall be mandatory for accreditation.[38]

So said Dr. John Porterfield, Director of the Joint Commission on Accreditation of Hospitals and the man in the middle of this power struggle.

In his inaugural address as President of the AHA, Mark Berke, Director, Mount Zion Hospital, San Francisco, spoke very frankly:

> We make a mistake, I believe, if we sweep the problem out of sight with glib statements about working together because our objectives are the same. Our objectives are not the same, although we travel down parallel roads that occasionally converge. The sooner we have the courage to look at the differences frankly and openly, the sooner we can begin to handle them and resolve them. The hospital can no longer

be regarded by physicians as simply a funnel through which the individual physician pours medical care into the individual patient. All the things society demands of us reject this approach.[39]

Indeed, the hospital-physician conflict is one of the principal and most difficult facts of life in the medical care picture today. It involves not only the professional, organizational, and financial relations of the physician to the hospital with which he is affiliated, and the role of the medical staff, but also the problem of the non-affiliated doctor and the hospital's responsibility to grant or deny staff privileges or perhaps provide them on a graded or limited basis. It also involves graduate medical education with the present confusion between service and training. The conflict creates formidable problems for hospital management, contributes to the rise in hospital costs, and inhibits the natural development of community health care planning.

The Battle of the Veto

The dramatic events of the last week of June 1970—the President's veto of the pending Hill-Burton legislation, providing $1.3 billion in grants and $1.5 billion in federally guaranteed and subsidized loans over a three-year period, followed by a decisive overriding of the veto in both houses of Congress—illustrate the extent to which the hospital has become both an object and a symbol of political and economic conflict.

The motives on both sides were clearly mixed and highly complex. They involved a constitutional tug-of-war between the executive and legislative branches of government, differences over allocation of national resources as between domestic and military needs, differences over how to fight inflation and recession, and so forth. However, the fact remains that the President chose this issue to challenge Congress and lost decisively, suggesting that the hospital is still a basically popular institution—one with deep roots in the American community as well as in the American health care economy.

*   *   *

Here, then, is Paradox Number Three: The hospital—which has emerged as the undisputed professional and technological center of the health care world, is our nearest approximation to a community health center, and still enjoys the confidence of most Americans—is prevented from playing the central coordinating role which its position logically dictates as a result of a combination of internal and external contradictions. Internally, the hospital has not been able to resolve the deep-rooted conflict between medical staff and lay administration, resulting in diffuse management and numerous inefficiencies. Externally, the hospital's role in the evolving health care system is challenged both by those who would turn the clock back to preinstitutional medicine and those who claim the center of the evolving system should not be the hospital but some type of primary care unit, apart from the hospital. Forced to carry multiple and ever-growing responsibilties, with these two major issues unresolved, the hospital's costs spiral ever upward and in turn add fuel to the fire of public criticism.

NOTES

1. *Darling v. Charleston Memorial Hospital,* 33 Ill. 2nd 326, 211 N.E. 2d. 253 (1965); *certiorari denied* 383 U.S. 946 (1966).

2. *Bing v. Thunig,* 2 N.Y. 2d 656, 143 N.E. 2d 3, 8 (1957).

3. *Goff v. Doctors' General Hospital of San José, Calif.* 333 P. 2d 29 (1958).

4. For review of the changing legal doctrines of negligence and corporate liability, as applied to hospitals, see, Somers, A. R., *Hospital Regulation: the Dilemma of Public Policy* (Princeton University, 1969), Chap. II.

5. U.S. Department of Health, Education, and Welfare, *Health, Education, and Welfare Trends,* 1964. p. 28.

6. *Hospitals, J.A.H.A.,* Guide Issue, Part 2, Aug. 1, 1967, p. 446. and Aug. 1, 1968, p. 438.

7. *Hospitals, J.A.H.A.,* Guide Issue, Part 2, Aug. 1, 1969, p. 475.

8. Reed, L. S. and Carr, W., Per capita expenditures for hospital care, 1966. U.S. Department of Health, Education, and Welfare, Social Security Administration, *Research and Statistics Note 13,* Aug. 1, 1969, p. 9.

9. U.S. Department of Health, Education, and Welfare, National Center for Health Statistics, *Regional Utilization of Short-Stay Hospitals, 1965,* USPHS Pub. No. 1000, Series 13, No. 5, June 1969, p. 2.

10. American Hospital Association, *Outpatient Health Care,* Report and Recommendations of a Conference on Hospital Outpatient Care (Chicago: the Association, 1969), p. 34.

11. *Hospitals, J.A.H.A.,* Guide Issue, Part 2, Aug. 1, 1958, p. 420, and Aug. 1, 1969, p. 497. Outpatient data are subject to some reporting errors, but orders of magnitude are correct.

12. Hospital Survey Committee, *Utilization Trends in Hospital Diagnostic Services,* Philadelphia, Jan. 1969, p. 13.

13. See, for example, articles in *Hospitals, J.A.H.A.,* July 1, 1969 (Special Issue, Health Services for the Poor); also Blue Cross Association, *Inquiry,* Mar. 1968 (Special Issue, Medical Care for Low-Income Families).

14. For the development of hospital planning, including the role of the Hill-Burton program, and some of the major problems now confronting the planning movement, see, Somers, *op. cit.* (Note 4), Chap. VII. Also, Somers, A. R., Goals into reality: the challenges of health planning. *Hospitals, J.A.H.A.,* Guide Issue, Part 1, Aug. 1, 1969, p. 41. Also, Libman, E. W., Why areawide planning falters. *Hospitals, J.A.H.A.,* July 16, 1969, p. 71.

15. American Hospital Association, *Statement on the Financial Requirements of Health Care Institutions and Services,* approved by House of Delegates, Feb. 12, 1969.

16. U.S. Department of Health, Education, and Welfare, Secretary's Advisory Committee on Hospital Effectiveness, *Report,* 1968.

17. Between 1950 and 1968 the average occupancy rate of community hospitals rose from 73.7 to 78.2. For the voluntary hospitals, the 1968 rate was 80.0; for state and local government and the proprietaries, 73.4. *Hospitals, J.A.H.A.,* Guide Issue, Part 2, Aug. 1, 1969, p. 475.

18. See, for example, Brown, R. E., Realigning the hospital system: emerging forces and evolving patterns, paper presented to Association of American Medical Colleges, Houston, Nov. 2, 1968.

19. Rice, D. P. and Cooper, B. S., National health expenditures, 1950-67, U.S. Department of Health, Education, and Welfare, *Soc. Secur. Bull.,* Jan. 1969, p. 12. Also, Rice and Cooper, National health expenditures, 1929-68, *Soc. Secur. Bull.,* Jan. 1970, p. 6.

20. *Hospitals, J.A.H.A.,* Guide Issue, Part 2, Aug. 1, 1969, p. 469. The concept of "expense per *adjusted* patient day" is used for the first time in the 1969 Guide Issue, replacing the obsolete "expense per patient day." Briefly, the new measure converts the number of outpatient visits into units roughly equivalent to an inpatient day in level of effort and combines these

"equivalent patient days" with the actual inpatient days. The new measure for 1968 is $5.58 lower than the old measure, which came to $61.38 (*Ibid.*, p. 475). It is a much more meaningful measure of total hospital costs in relation to output.

21. *Hospitals, J.A.H.A.*, May 16, 1970, p. 48.

22. U.S. Department of Labor, Bureau of Labor Statistics, *Consumer Price Index*, Feb. 1970. 1957-1959=100.

23. Tolchin, M., The changing city: a medical challenge. *New York Times*, June 2, 1969.

24. Anderson, A. C., Executive Director, Strong Memorial Hospital, Nov. 20, 1969.

25. Nearly two-thirds of all short-term hospitals had less than 100 beds, as late as 1965, and more than 82 percent had less than 200. U.S. Department of Health, Education, and Welfare, National Center for Health Statistics, *Patients Discharged from Short-Stay Hospitals, 1965*, USPHS Pub. No. 1000, Series 13, No. 4, Dec. 1968, p. 2. This is probably related to other findings of the Hospital Discharge Survey: More than one-third of all United States short-stay hospitals are in the South, and the average number of beds per hospital—178—was higher in the Northeast than in the North Central states—131; the South—98; or the West— 83. *Regional Utilization of Short-Stay Hospitals, 1965*, USPHS Pub. 1000, Series 13, No. 5, June 1969. p. 1.

26. *Hospitals, J.A.H.A.*, Guide Issue, Part 2, Aug. 1, 1969, p. 468.

27. Romano, J., And leave for the unknown. *J. Amer. Med. Assn.* Oct. 26, 1964, p. 283.

28. *New York Times*, Feb. 27, 1970.

29. *New York Times*, May 27, 1970.

30. *Mod. Hosp.*, Dec. 1969. p. 93. For various views as to the significance of the new chains, see several articles in this issue. Also, *Mod. Hosp.*, March 1969. Also, Owens, A., Can the profit motive save our hospitals? *Med. Econ.*, Mar. 30, 1970. Also, Big business in medical facilities. *Amer. Med. News*, May 11, 1970. For a related development, see, Earle, P. W., The nursing home industry. *Hospitals, J.A.H.A.*, Feb. 16, 1970, p. 45, and Mar. 1, 1970, p. 60.

31. Tolchin, *op. cit.*

32. Duff, R. S. and Hollingshead, A. B., *Sickness and Society* (New York: Harper & Row, 1968).

33. Hubbard, W. N., Jr., *Med. World News*, Mar. 31, 1967.

34. Geiger, H. J., Health and social change: the urban crisis, Lowell Lecture, Boston, Feb. 12, 1968, p. 13 (mimeo.).

35. Stewart, W. H., The next fifty years, paper delivered to American Institute of Planners, Oct. 5, 1967, p. 10 (mimeo.).

36. For discussion of the conflict in public criticism and public regulation and a review of the principal forms of regulation now in effect. see, Somers, *Hospital Regulation, op. cit.* (Note 4).

37. *Med. Econ.*, Aug. 4, 1969, p. 38.

38. *Med. Econ.*, Nov. 24, 1969, p. 231.

39. Incoming President Mark Berke's inaugural address. *Hospitals, J.A.H.A.*, Mar. 16, 1970, p. 65.

Chapter 4

RECENT DEVELOPMENTS IN FINANCING*

An ironic element in that increase [in medical care costs] has been that every forward-looking reform for erasing the sometimes catastrophic burden of illness for low- and middle-income families—Medicare, Medicaid, and employer-financed insurance through Blue Cross and Blue Shield—has had the perverse effect of spurring the upsurge in overall costs.

New York Times
Editorial (August 17, 1969)

The major recent developments in the financing of medical care stem from the scientific, technological, professional, and demographic developments discussed in Chapters 1, 2, and 3. The highly trained medical specialists and the new instrumentation, the facilities to house it, and the skilled manpower to operate it are inevitably expensive. Hospitals are expensive both to build and to operate. Virtually all the demographic trends we have noted result in greater demand for medical care and greater expense—both over the life of any given individual and to the nation in any given year.

The $64 Billion Question

The result has been a spectacular increase in both family and national expenditures for health. For the nation as a whole, health expenditures (not counting medical and health education) rose from $13 billion in 1950 to $57 billion in 1968 (Table 1, next page). During the same period, the proportion of the gross national product going for health care rose from 4.5 percent to 6.6 percent, an increase of 47 percent.

The rate of increase, far from leveling off, has been accelerating. Between 1950 and 1966, the average annual rise in total expenditures was 8.2 percent. From 1966 to 1967, the rise was 12.6 percent; for 1967 to 1968, 12.7 percent. At this rate, the figure for 1969 will be about $64.5 billion and for 1970, about $73 billion. We shall exceed $100 billion and approach 8 to 10 percent of GNP within a few years.

*In the interest of brevity, the discussion in this chapter has been limited almost entirely to operating costs. However, the same general trends apply to the problem of capital costs. Here, too, the burden had to be spread over the entire population by means of government grants and loans, philanthropic donations, and increasingly through third-party reimbursement, as is now the case under Medicare and most Blue Cross hospital contracts. In this area, also, prices and costs have increased astronomically.

Table 1: Amount and Percentage Distribution of National Health Expenditures by Type of Expenditure, Selected Years, 1950-68

Type of expenditure	1950	1960	1965	1967	1968
	AMOUNTS (IN MILLIONS)				
Total	$12,867	$26,973	$40,591	$50,655	$57,103
Health services and supplies	11,910	25,263	37,210	46,885	53,078
Hospital care	3,845	9,044	13,520	17,946	20,751
Federal facilities	728	1,221	1,600	1,877	2,151
State and local facilities	1,175	2,827	3,990	5,054	6,039
Nongovernmental facilities	1,942	4,996	7,930	11,016	12,562
Physicians' services	2,755	5,684	8,745	10,163	11,562
Dentists' services	975	1,977	2,808	3,186	3,612
Other professional services	395	862	1,038	1,447	1,342
Drugs and drug sundries	1,730	3,657	4,850	5,569	6,149
Eyeglasses and appliances	490	776	1,230	1,584	1,718
Nursing home care	142	526	1,328	1,858	2,282
Expenses for prepayment and administration	300	863	1,297	1,777	1,847
Government public health activities	361	412	696	914	969
Other health services	917	1,462	1,698	2,441	2,846
Research and medical facilities construction	957	1,710	3,381	3,770	4,025
Research	117	662	1,469	1,775	1,765
Construction	840	1,048	1,912	1,995	2,260
Publicly owned	496	443	521	628	694
Privately owned	344	605	1,391	1,367	1,566

PERCENTAGE DISTRIBUTION

Total	100.0	100.0	100.0	100.0	100.0
Health services and supplies	92.6	93.7	91.7	92.6	93.0
Hospital care	29.9	33.5	33.3	35.4	36.3
Federal facilities	5.7	4.5	3.9	3.7	3.8
State and local facilities	9.1	10.5	9.8	10.0	10.6
Nongovernmental facilities	15.1	18.5	19.5	21.7	22.0
Physicians' services	21.4	21.1	21.5	20.1	20.2
Dentists' services	7.6	7.3	6.9	6.3	6.3
Other professional services	3.1	3.2	2.6	2.9	2.4
Drugs and drug sundries	13.4	13.6	11.9	11.0	10.8
Eyeglasses and appliances	3.8	2.9	3.0	3.1	3.0
Nursing home care	1.1	2.0	3.3	3.7	4.0
Expenses for prepayment and administration	2.3	3.2	3.2	3.5	3.2
Government public health activities	2.8	1.5	1.7	1.8	1.7
Other health services	7.1	5.4	4.2	4.8	5.0
Research and medical facilities construction	7.4	6.3	8.3	7.4	7.0
Research	.9	2.5	3.6	3.5	3.1
Construction	6.5	3.9	3.6	3.5	4.0
Publicly owned	3.9	1.6	1.3	1.2	1.2
Privately owned	2.7	2.2	3.4	2.7	2.7
Total expenditures as a percent of gross national product	4.5	5.4	5.9	6.4	6.6
Total expenditures per capita	$165	$197	$245	$267	$280

Source: Rice, D. P., and Cooper, B. S., National health expenditures, 1950-67, *Soc. Secur. Bull.*, Jan. 1969, p. 12; National health expenditures, 1929-68, *Ibid.*, Jan. 1970, pp. 12, 15.

Along with the overall rise has come a substantial shift in the distribution of expenditures among different types of services reflecting, primarily, the changing technology of health care. Until the end of the 1930s, physicians' services accounted for the largest single share of health care costs. By 1940, hospitals had moved to first place in the cost table, and they have steadily increased their portion ever since. As noted in Chapter 3, in 1968, hospitals took 40 percent of the health care dollar (including 4 percent for construction). As a result of the extraordinary rise in hospital costs, most of the other categories have declined proportionately. Physicians in private practice dropped from 21 percent in 1950 to 20 percent, dentists from 8 to 6 percent (Table 1). Among the few categories that increased was nursing home care, only one percent in 1950 and 4 percent in 1968. Medical research, less than one percent in 1950, moved up to 3 percent.

The principal factors in the rise in health care expenditures are charted on the next page. The data apply only to expenditures for personal health care, eliminating research, construction, the net cost of health insurance, and public health measures. But personal health care is the area where the most dramatic rises have taken place. Population growth accounted for 18 percent, but this factor is readily placed in perspective by comparing per capita expenditures for the various years as shown on Table 1. For 1950, the amount was $165; for 1968, $280.[1]

Quality improvements, greater use, and other factors accounted for just over one-third of the overall rise, while nearly half resulted from price increases or inflation.[2]

However measured, the rise in the price of health services since World War II has been startling. Of course, prices have been going up everywhere. Price increases in the general economy have contributed to the inflation in health care prices. But the differential between the general and health care price increases during the past two decades has been pronounced and persistent. According to the Bureau of Labor Statistics (BLS), health care prices rose 155 percent from 1946 to 1969, while the general cost of living rose 88 percent. The average annual rise for health care was 4.2 percent; for the general index, 2.8 percent. The major factor in the health care rise was the price of a hospital room, which, as noted in Chapter 3, was nearly 300 percent higher in mid-1970 than it was a decade earlier. Rising physician fees have also contributed substantially (Chapter 1).

For years, it was optimistically said that this was all part of a catching-up process, since health care prices had fallen behind other prices during the Great Depression and hospital wages were making up their lag behind other wage scales. After a reasonable period, so the argument ran, we could expect a leveling out, and the movement of health care prices would then be consistent with other price movements. The prediction has proved invalid. In recent years the differential has actually widened. The year 1969 was an exception because general prices experienced an extraordinary inflation of 5.4 percent. Even then health care prices rose more sharply, 6.9 percent. In the three-month period ending May 1970, health care costs rose 2.2 percent; all items, 1.6 percent.

The single most obvious result of the rising costs and prices has been the development of new methods for paying them. This was an absolute necessity.

[1] For this and succeeding notes in this chapter, see page 71.

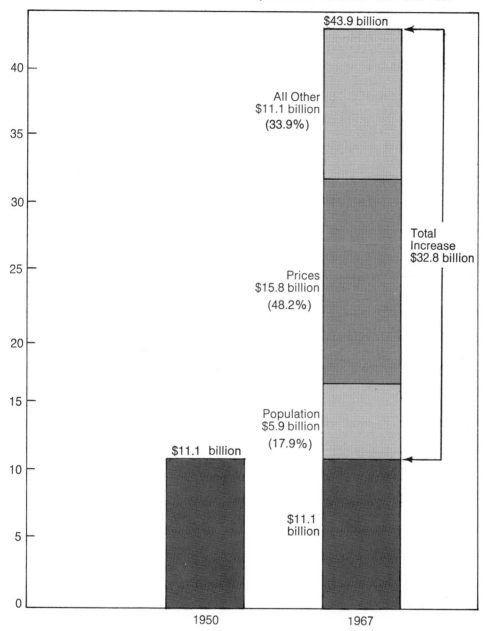

Factors in the Rise in Health Care Expenditures Between 1950 and 1967

Source: Rice, D. P. and Cooper, B. S. *Soc. Secur. Bull.* Jan. 1969, p. 14.

Individuals and single families could not possibly meet the current cost of serious illness. Even routine hospitalization is prohibitive for many families. One midwestern hospital reported that, between 1966 and 1970, the average bill for a new baby (hospital bill only) went up more than 100 percent: from $234 to $493 for a routine delivery, from $377 to $763 for a cesarean section. According to the BLS, the total cost of having and outfitting an infant has risen 35 percent since 1965. All of this adds up to a total price tag of $1500 for a perfectly normal baby. If the birth is complicated—premature or cesarean—it is likely to be $2500, even higher in New York City or California.[3]

Private health insurance and tax-supported programs were society's response to this need, and we are fortunate indeed that the insurance industry, both the nonprofit and for-profit varieties, and the Congress have risen to this challenge as well as they have. It is only because most Americans now have most of their hospital bills and a substantial part of their doctors' bills paid by such third parties that the new technological health care economy has been able to continue to grow and the health needs and expectations of the American people could be translated into effective demand.

The history of third-party financing in the United States has been stormy and controversial from the outset. This is not only because the financial stakes are so high—billions of dollars are involved annually—but, even more important, because many of the more sophisticated providers and consumers see in the financing programs a major key to future control of the entire industry. Following are brief résumés of major historical developments with respect to private health insurance and the major public programs.

Private Health Insurance

Insurance companies have developed an active and growing interest in the costs of care, increased efficiency in providing care, community planning for health services, peer review, the organization of health care, and the quality of the care which their benefits purchase. They are aware that in significant respects the insurer stands in the position of a trustee for its insureds, charged with responsibility to represent their best interests as consumers of health care.

J. F. FOLLMANN JR.
Pension and Welfare News (February 1969)

At first unsophisticated about the need for government programs to help the disadvantaged, carriers are now learning to work with government. . . . Perhaps the fundamental flaw is an excess of publicly unrewarding competition among carriers vis-à-vis largely uncompetitive producers of services. Health care is involved in what often seem to be contradictory values of access, dignity, innovation, variety, and uniformity. If these values are to be properly balanced, the remedy lies in stronger internal and external disciplines for the entire industry.

WALTER J. MCNERNEY
Private Health Insurance and Medical Care (1968)

The significant role played by private health insurance in the United States, in contrast to almost all other nations, may be attributed to a combination of affluence, our marked preference for private as opposed to governmental enterprise, the ingenuity and energy of the principal carriers, and a fortuitous "shotgun marriage" between medical care and industrial relations in the 1940s and 1950s.[4]

Starting from near zero, in 1929, when the first local prepayment plan was launched in Dallas, with only a few hundred school teachers, enrollment has grown to the point where approximately 80 percent of the population now has some degree of coverage. Involved in this phenomenal 40-year growth were all kinds of institutions—nonprofit plans such as Blue Cross and Blue Shield; commercial insurance, both mutual and stock companies; and a heterogeneous group known as "independents" including consumer-controlled plans such as the Health Insurance Plan of Greater New York (HIP), Group Health Insurance, Inc., of New York and New Jersey, Group Health Association of Washington, D.C., and Group Health Cooperative of Puget Sound, provider-controlled plans such as the Ross-Loos Medical Group of Los Angeles and the San Joaquin County (California) Medical Foundation, plans controlled by labor or management such as the United Mine Workers Welfare and Retirement Fund, and numerous "health and welfare funds" in many of our major cities.

One of the most important plans in the country, the Kaiser Foundation Health Plan, virtually defies classification. Starting as an industrial health program for Kaiser industry employees, before and during World War II, it has grown to a vast network of community hospitals, clinics, and medical groups, and about two million members in California, Washington, Oregon, and Hawaii, and since 1969 in Cleveland and in Denver.[5]

Underlying this fascinating diversity, however, were certain basic and common factors: on the one hand, the medical profession's adamant opposition to government-financed medical care programs; on the other hand, the unrelenting pressure of organized labor for some type of third-party financing mechanism, and the ability of United States industry to absorb or to pass on, in price increases, a large part of the total cost. It was entirely coincidental that the doctors' successful campaigns against public health insurance during the late 1930s and the 1940s coincided with the vast expansion of organized labor and collective bargaining. But the implications were great.

From the end of World War II, the growth of private health insurance and of industrial "health and welfare" plans were inextricably interrelated. Enlightened management's increasing concern for "human relations" in industry, the wartime wage stabilization program with its encouragement of "fringe benefits," and the effect of National Labor Relations Board and United States Supreme Court decisions in making such benefits a routine matter for collective bargaining were all compelling factors. Most of the significant advances in insurance enrollment and in benefit coverage have been associated with collective bargaining agreements in major industries such as auto, steel, mining, building trades, longshoring, men's and women's apparel, etc.

Achievements and Problems

Estimates of the civilian population with some private health insurance coverage at the end of 1968 vary from 77 to 85 percent, depending on the method of counting. The higher figure comes from the Health Insurance Association of America, spokesman for the insurance industry;[6] the lower figure from the United States Department of Health, Education, and Welfare, which utilizes, among other estimating techniques, household surveys conducted by the National Center for Health Statistics.[7]

For persons under 65, the 1968 estimates from HEW are 80 percent with some hospital coverage, 77 percent with some surgical coverage, 46 percent with some coverage of doctors' office and home calls, 43 percent for out-of-hospital prescribed drugs, down to 3 percent with dental benefits. Most of the out-of-hospital benefits, however, are provided under "major medical" policies that allow benefits only after payment of an out-of-pocket deductible and with an additional coinsurance factor. In any one year only a small proportion of covered persons would have any part of their expenses for these items reimbursed.

Among those 65 and over, the HEW estimates (1968) are 49 percent with some hospital benefits, in addition to Medicare, and 47 percent with some surgical benefits. Before Medicare it was estimated that about 60 percent of the aged had some sort of insurance protection. The large number who have continued their private insurance reflects the continuing fear of heavy medical expenses and willingness to pay for as full protection as can be obtained.

As with the younger population, most of the aged also have only inhospital benefits. The proportion with nursing home or home health benefits is low—11 to 15 percent. Furthermore, since major medical policies, which provide almost all the coverage of doctors' office and home visits, uniformly exclude coverage of physician services for physical examinations and health checkups, it follows that almost all of the private insurance held by the aged is for the care of illness and very little gives any coverage for prevention.

In short, some 30 to 40 million Americans have no health insurance whatsoever, and as many as 60 million more under the age of 65 have coverage which is, in the words of Wilbur Cohen, former Secretary of HEW, "grossly inadequate or at least less than that provided to the aged under Medicare."[8] Moreover, the distribution of health insurance coverage is badly skewed. Practically all the rich have insurance. But among the poor, about two-thirds have none. As a result, among people aged 25 to 64 who die, some 45 to 50 percent have neither hospital nor surgical coverage.

The 1968 distribution of total gross enrollment among the three groups of insurance organizations—the "Blue" Plans, the insurance companies, and the independents—for the different benefits and for the two age groups, is shown in Table 2 (opposite). With respect to the aged, the "Blue" Plans have been relatively more successful in selling coverage complementary to Medicare, although the difference with respect to hospital care is now minimal.

Among those under 65, however, the insurance companies have dramatically outdistanced the "Blues," especially for the newer out-of-hospital benefits. This results primarily from the wide sale of major medical policies, which now account for over 60 percent of all insurance company coverages. The only area where the "Blues" still lead is nursing home care.

Table 2: Percentage Distribution of Gross Enrollment Among Carriers, 1968

Age group and type of plan	Hospital care	Physician services				Dental care	Pre-scribed drugs (out of hospital)	Private duty nursing	Visiting nurse service	Nursing home care
		Surgical services	In-hospital visits	X-ray and labora-tory examina-tions	Office and home visits					
Total, all ages	100.0	100.0	100.0	100.0	100.0	100.0	100.0	100.0	100.0	100.0
Blue Cross-Blue Shield	36.4	35.7	41.9	27.2	18.1	.6	17.9	20.8	25.5	63.8
Insurance companies	59.8	59.5	52.4	64.7	73.8	53.7	77.6	74.1	68.3	28.8
Group policies	39.3	43.6	43.7	57.9	66.4	52.8	71.4	67.8	62.5	16.3
Individual policies	20.5	15.9	8.7	6.8	7.4	.8	6.2	6.3	5.8	12.5
Independent plans	3.8	4.8	5.7	8.0	8.0	45.7	4.5	5.1	6.1	7.5
Under age 65, total	100.0	100.0	100.0	100.0	100.0	100.0	100.0	100.0	100.0	100.0
Blue Cross-Blue Shield	35.7	34.7	40.8	26.3	17.5	.6	17.5	20.9	25.3	61.0
Insurance companies	60.6	60.5	53.6	65.8	74.6	53.7	78.2	74.2	68.8	31.8
Group policies	40.6	44.9	45.0	58.8	67.1	52.9	71.9	67.9	62.9	17.7
Individual policies	20.0	15.6	8.6	7.0	7.5	.8	6.2	6.3	5.9	14.0
Independent plans	3.7	4.8	5.6	7.9	7.9	45.6	4.4	5.0	6.0	7.2
Age 65 and over, total	100.0	100.0	100.0	100.0	100.0	100.0	100.0	100.0	100.0	100.0
Blue Cross-Blue Shield	49.1	54.0	62.8	49.6	37.3	—	30.2	17.5	34.9	85.8
Insurance companies	47.0	40.8	30.5	38.1	50.3	49.0	60.0	69.8	53.7	4.7
Group policies	17.5	19.8	20.7	34.7	45.9	49.0	54.8	63.7	49.1	4.7
Individual policies	29.5	21.0	9.7	3.3	4.4	—	5.2	6.1	4.7	—
Independent plans	3.9	5.1	6.7	12.3	12.3	51.0	9.8	12.7	11.4	9.6

Source: Reed, L. S., Private health insurance, 1968: enrollment, coverage, and financial experience, *Soc. Secur. Bull.*, Dec. 1969, p. 24.

The independents provide a very small percentage of the total although they show greater strength in the out-of-hospital categories—reflecting the emphasis most of these plans place on comprehensive coverage. They account for over half the enrollment for dental benefits.[9]

The value of all these benefits depends on the extent to which they actually meet health care costs. Despite a long-run gradual improvement in the benefit/expenditure ratio, in 1968 insurance benefits still met only 36 percent of the total expenditures by private consumers (Table 3, below).[10]

Table 3: Proportion of Consumer Expenditures Paid for Through Health Insurance, Selected Years, 1950-68*

Year	Total	Hospital care	Physician services	Other types of care
1950	12.1	34.6	12.0	†
1955	21.5	51.8	25.0	†
1960	27.7	63.7	30.0	1.3
1961	29.9	66.2	32.7	1.7
1962	30.9	68.2	33.0	1.9
1963	31.7	67.2	33.6	2.1
1964	31.5	68.1	32.2	2.3
1965	32.4	70.2	32.7	2.5
1966	32.0	67.6	33.8	2.8
1967	33.1	70.1	36.2	3.8
1968	35.7	73.7	38.4	4.2

*Excludes net cost of insurance—the difference between premiums and benefit expenditures.
†Included in physician services.
Source: Reed, L. S., Private health insurance, 1968: enrollment, coverage, and financial experience, *Soc. Secur. Bull.,* Dec. 1969, p. 35.

Only in the area of hospital care has private insurance achieved really significant benefit coverage—nearly three-fourths of consumer expenditures. With respect to doctors' bills, insurance met only a little over 38 percent of the total in 1968. Nor is there any basis for anticipating significant progress in the near future. The slow rise with respect to all types of out-of-hospital benefits is particularly discouraging since this is the area of greatest potential economy.

The 1968 financial experience of private health insurance organizations is summarized in Table 4 (opposite). They had a total subscription or premium income of $13 billion; paid out 88 percent, over $11 billion, in benefits; used 14.8 percent for operating expenses; and had a net underwriting loss of nearly 3 percent. The only segments of the industry that appear to be thriving financially are the dental societies, whose plans produced a net surplus of 11 percent, and Blue Shield, with a 5 percent surplus. Losses were heaviest—nearly 7 percent of premium income—in the insurance company group business, where it was at least partially offset by investment income (although data on this are not available), as well as by profits from more lucrative types of group insurance frequently sold in the same package. Blue Cross sustained a net loss of 2 percent.

It is evident that, aside from the notoriously inefficient insurance company individual policies (in this category operating expenses or "retention" consumed nearly half of income and, even so, the companies failed to show a profit), there is not much room for administrative improvement. Private health insurance has, in

Table 4: Financial Experience of Private Health Insurance Organizations, 1968
(Amounts in Millions)

Type of plan	Total Income	Subscription or premium income	Claims expense		Operating expense		Net under-writing gain		Net income	
			Amount	Percent of premium income	Amount	Percent of premium income	Amount	Percent of premium income	Amount	Percent of total income
Total	*	$12,860.6	$11,309.6	87.9	$1,907.2	14.8	−$356.2	−2.8	*	......
Blue Cross-Blue Shield	$5,285.1	5,187.1	4,840.6	93.3	375.1	7.2	−28.6	−.5	$69.5	1.3
Blue Cross	3,728.9	3,665.0	3,529.2	96.3	208.6	5.7	−72.8	−2.0	−8.9	−.2
Blue Shield	1,556.2	1,522.1	1,311.4	86.2	166.5	10.9	44.2	2.9	78.4	5.0
Insurance companies	*	6,933.0	5,791.0	83.5	1,488.8	21.5	−346.8	−5.0	*	......
Group policies	*	5,159.0	4,841.0	93.8	660.4	12.8	−342.4	−6.6	*	......
Individual policies	*	1,774.0	950.0	53.6	828.4	46.7	−4.4	−.2	*	......
Independent plans	740.5	740.5	678.0	91.6	43.3	5.8	19.2	2.6	19.2	2.6
Community	310.0	310.0	290.0	93.5	20.0	6.5	0	0	*	......
Employer-employee-union	380.0	380.0	345.0	90.8	20.0	5.3	15.0	3.9	15.0	3.9
Private group clinic	16.0	16.0	14.5	90.6	1.0	6.3	.5	3.1	.5	3.1
Dental society	34.5	34.5	28.5	82.6	2.3	6.7	3.7	10.7	3.7	10.7

*Data not available.

Source: Reed, L. S., Private health insurance, 1968: enrollment, coverage, and financial experience, *Soc. Secur. Bull.*, Dec. 1969, p. 31.

effect, become largely a "cost plus" operation except that, ironically, for most of the industry, the "plus" has become a "minus." It may be significant that the smaller independent plans, with their emphasis on out-of-hospital benefits, appear to be at least holding their own.

Since 1968 the pressure on the carriers has continued to mount relentlessly. In mid-1969, Blue Cross of Massachusetts reported that it had paid $87,000 in one case, a woman with a rare but usually curable polyneuritis, and the case was not yet closed.[11] Although this was reported to be the highest amount paid by any Blue Cross Plan for a single case, claims of $25,000 to $50,000 are no longer unusual.

Unlike the insurance companies, however, Blue Cross Plans, in most states, must obtain the approval of state insurance commissioners for rate increases. In at least two states, New York and New Jersey, the increases requested in 1969, averaging 49.5 percent in New York and 44.3 percent in New Jersey, precipitated bitter political battles. The press, the politicians (especially in New York City), the unions, and millions of individual Blue Cross members waxed indignant and swore publicly and privately throughout the summer. The City of New York requested a court order directing the State Insurance Department to show cause why the increases should not be barred. The city also threatened to set up its own "Blue Cross" on a self-insured basis.

Despite all the tumult and the shouting, however, no one had any effective remedy for the underlying inflation in provider costs. The whole bitter drama was marked by a pervasive atmosphere of futility and frustration. Faced with the undeniable fact that the plans could not stay in business without a substantial rise in premium income, the insurance commissioners had little choice except to grant most of what the plans were asking. New York Blue Cross got 43.3 percent; New Jersey an emergency 28.5 in December and another 21.9 in May 1970. It was understood that a further increase would be required by mid-1971.

A particularly poignant casualty of the current inflation was the long-standing Montefiore Medical Group, HIP's showcase affiliate since the start of the plan in 1947. The hospital claimed that it could not provide services for the payment HIP was able to make for its members. HIP claimed it could not pay more. A 40 percent subscriber rate increase had already been put into effect early in 1969.

By the summer of 1970, the problems facing Blue Cross in many parts of the country were reaching crisis proportions. The honeymoon between Blue Cross and the hospitals was generally at an end. Forced by subscriber pressure and state legislatures to put the screws on hospitals, Blue Cross was even fighting implementation of the new AHA reimbursement policy (Chapter 3). Presumably the long-run advantage of putting more teeth into planning was outweighed by the immediate cost of a capital factor based on current-cost replacement and sharing the cost of indigent care. In several eastern states, the renewal of Blue Cross-hospital contracts was being approached with growing hostility on both sides.

Meanwhile, the era of relatively good feeling between Blue Cross and the commercial carriers, the product of the phenomenal post-war growth enjoyed by all, was also coming to an end. In several states Blue Cross was being sued by insurance companies as an "unlawful monopoly"; in others, the carriers were stepping up pressure on state legislatures to revoke Blue Cross exemption from the usual premium tax. In turn, Blue Cross was demanding that the insurance companies be brought under greater state regulation. In the growing atmosphere of tension and pessimism more and more carriers, as well as hospitals, were looking, anxiously if somewhat surreptitiously, to government to provide a way out, a posture already held by numerous consumer groups (Chapter 8).

In the growing disappointment over the inability of the private carriers and health insurance funds to adequately insure the entire population and to meet the growing crisis in health care costs, however, it would be a serious error to over-look their many impressive achievements.

First, there is the basic fact that millions of people have obtained access to good medical care for the first time. For example, the United Mine Workers Welfare and Retirement Fund reported a 30 percent gain in the average life expectancy of bituminous coal miners between 1946, when the Fund began, and 1967. At the earlier date, miners died at a median age of 57.4, more than 8 years earlier than the average United States male. In 1967, the average age of a miner at death was 74.7, over 6 years older than the general average.[12] Allowing for the possibility of some exaggeration and the fact that health benefits were not the only cause of the increased longevity, nevertheless the improvement must be at least partially attributed to the union health program. The same, to varying degrees, could be said of many other insurance or prepayment plans.

Second, it has been possible, by spreading the risks and costs of care, to develop a much broader and stronger financial base for our rapidly expanding medical care economy. The fact that the private sector has been unable to cope adequately with the special problems of the aged and the poor should not obscure those areas where they have proved both innovative and successful.

In a sense the carriers have been the victim of their own success. Perhaps it was too easy to translate relatively modest contributions from thousands of employers and millions of employees into $50-, $60-, and even $100-a-day hospital payments. There are those who fault the carriers for not controlling these costs more effec-tively. The fact is that they were unable to do so, an inability that Medicare and Medicaid have similarly demonstrated. This latter should give pause to those who believe that national health insurance would provide a magic instrument of control.

Innovations and Improvements

Among the most innovative programs, one thinks immediately of prepaid group practice, associated with Kaiser, HIP, Group Health Cooperative of Puget Sound, and others. The obstacles faced by these organizations, especially in their early days, were very great. Not all have been successful in overcoming them, but several have been, spectacularly so. What has come to be known as the "Kaiser Formula" can now be accepted as an experiment that has fully proved itself over a period of 26 years.

The essential ingredients of this formula, as defined by the medical director of its Portland Clinic, include (1) prepayment, usually by monthly dues; (2) group practice; (3) a unified medical center, including both hospital and satellite clinics; (4) voluntary enrollment, based on the choice of two or more different kinds of health plans; (5) payment of physicians and hospitals on the basis of capitation or fixed fees per time period for each enrollee, regardless of the amount of care provided; and (6) coverage of the full spectrum of comprehensive care, starting with prevention.[13]

Nor has success been confined to prepaid group practice. Group Health Insurance (GHI), with 1.3 million enrollees in New York and New Jersey, and the much smaller San Joaquin County Medical Foundation, operated by the medical society in that county, have both demonstrated that something approaching comprehensive coverage can be provided even without group practice, without a hospital base, and without capitation payment.

Despite these differences, however, there are some basic similarities among these programs. The common ingredients in Kaiser and GHI, for example, can probably be identified as the *sine qua non* of a successful health insurance program today:

1. Both view their responsibility primarily as providers of health care, not just as conduits for medical expense dollars.

2. Both assume responsibility for the cost and, to a lesser extent, the quality of such care. GHI doctors are all in private independent practice but they must accept a fixed-fee schedule without income limits, and this has been maintained despite pressure from Medicare and other sources. GHI quality controls are not so direct as under Kaiser but their claims are constantly scrutinized for appropriateness as well as price.

3. Both plans are distinguished by strong, independent management, making full use of computer capability and other modern managerial tools.

Blue Cross, through the Blue Cross Association and individual plans, has long been in the forefront of efforts to strengthen private health insurance.[14] In its 1970 Member Hospital Reimbursement Formula, the Associated Hospital Service of New York, the largest Blue Cross Plan, has introduced, in accordance with New York State's 1969 Hospital Cost Control Law, several important new features, including a productivity incentive payment, a utilization-control incentive payment, and a trusteed community pool of depreciation funds. A few Blue Cross Plans are underwriting prepaid group practice and other innovative programs.

The commercial insurance industry, long a bastion of conservatism, has now become a champion of progressive developments in the delivery system, developments aimed at both better cost controls and more comprehensive coverage.[15] Several companies are underwriting prepaid group practice experiments.

Perhaps the most interesting program in the entire field of private health insurance is the Federal Employees Health Benefits Program (FEP). This huge plan, which has been in existence for 10 years and is successfully insuring over eight million persons, including nearly 450,000 retirees, constitutes a creative, pragmatic mix of public and private initiative.[16] Indeed, it is difficult to be sure of the correct way to classify it, whether public or private. In the various federal reports, however (for example, Table 1), it is classified as private, even though it is statutory, since its benefits are entirely underwritten by private carriers and the government participates principally in the role of employer.

Under FEP, federal employees choose, at specified intervals, from among a number of different types of carriers and different benefit packages carrying different price tags. There are strict limitations on the number and qualifications of carriers. The 38 currently approved organizations include a governmentwide Blue Cross-Blue Shield Plan, a governmentwide consortium of insurance companies administered by Aetna Life and Casualty, a group of employee union plans, a group of comprehensive group practice plans including Kaiser and HIP, and a few comprehensive individual practice plans such as GHI and the San Joaquin Foundation Plan. All are permitted to sell the best program they can underwrite. Most sell a "low" option and a "high" option, providing broader benefits at a higher price. Enrollment under the high options has steadily increased since the program started, until today about 85 percent of enrollees are so covered.

All plans provide a wide range of benefits, exceeding by a substantial margin the insurance available to most Americans at comparable prices. Under the high options, the following benefits are generally available, although with some variation as to adequacy: inpatient hospitalization, most physician services, most hospital ambulatory services, psychiatric care, prescribed drugs, and some appliances. The principal gaps involve physical checkups, dental care, and long-term care.

Premiums vary widely. Originally the government, as employer, contributed to all plans an amount equal to half the premium of the low-option Aetna plan. This resulted in the government paying about 38 percent of total costs. The difference between the government contribution and the actual premium of the plan selected by the employee is paid by him, thus providing a brake on rising costs and an incentive to intercarrier competition. In recent years, the rising costs of all health insurance resulted in a decline in the government proportion to 24 percent. Congress is currently debating how much to raise the federal contribution—probably to 40 to 50 percent.

The program is administered by the U.S. Civil Service Commission, which approves the various benefit packages and the prices charged for them, conducts the various "open enrollment" periods including approval of the informational material distributed by the competing carriers, collects the required contributions, and funnels them to the participating carriers.

The distribution of enrollees among the various plans has been relatively stable, although with some significant changes, over the years. Following are the percentages for 1960 and for March 1970:

	1960	*1970*
Blue Cross-Blue Shield	54.2	60.8
Aetna	26.9	18.0
Employee plans	13.2	14.6
Group practice plans	4.2	4.9
Individual practice plans	1.5	1.7

It must be kept in mind, of course, that the two latter categories are local and not available in many parts of the country.

One of the interesting aspects of FEP is the opportunity it affords to compare utilization of health services under the different types of insurance. Consistently, the comprehensive plans have demonstrated lower hospital use, in terms of both admissions and days, than the more conventional programs. For example, the rates for nonmaternity inpatient hospitalization under the different plans, both options, in 1966 were as follows:

	Utilizers per 1000 covered persons	Hospital days per 1000 covered persons
Blue Cross-Blue Shield	98	876
Aetna	85	884
Employee plans	93	808
Group practice plans	46	408
Individual practice plans	71	499

The total cost of FEP has increased over the years from $343 million, or $59 per capita, in 1962 to $826 million, or $104 per capita, in 1969. While some significant benefit improvements have taken place during this period, clearly FEP has not been immune to the general inflation. Nevertheless, $104 is still low for the coverage provided, and satisfaction among FEP enrollees is generally high. This is a program to be studied carefully in any movement toward national health insurance.

Rather than issue either a blanket condemnation or a total endorsement of private health insurance, it is essential to sort out the different experiences of different carriers, to distinguish the successful from the unsuccessful, and to seek ways of assimilating and generalizing the positive. Among the reforms that have been suggested are:

1. Elimination or reduction of the usual statutory limitations on Blue Cross and Blue Shield benefit coverage, including merger of the two programs.

2. Establishment of minimum state benefit standards for all carriers, with special emphasis on out-of-hospital benefits.

3. Repeal of all state laws restricting the establishment of prepaid group practice plans.

4. A requirement that, in all states where such plans now exist, tax-exempt employee benefit plans include, in their health benefits, a prepaid group practice option.

5. Provision in state laws for the self-employed and other individuals who lack access to group coverage to be treated as groups in order to obtain the benefit of group rates.

6. Compulsory coverage of part-time and temporarily employed workers, and of those temporarily laid off.

7. Noncancellability of policies in effect for a year and convertibility from group to individual coverage at equitable rates.

8. Public subsidy to carriers sponsoring experimental programs, such as prepaid group practice.

9. Prohibition of duplicate benefits, especially for hospital confinement.

10. Prohibition or strict control on mail-order insurance.

11. Reduction in the number of carriers, from the present 1700 or more, to a comparatively few with the size and administrative strength to match the problems.

Some of these proposals have been recommended in recent HEW reports, including the National Conference on Private Health Insurance (1967), the Secretary's Advisory Committee on Hospital Effectiveness (1968), and the Secretary's Task Force on Medicaid and Related Programs (1970).

The final result of pursuing this approach to its logical conclusion would be designation of a limited number of carriers as "chosen instruments"—operating for profit but under strict public regulation, which might or might not permit competition. The transition from such regulated private health insurance to certain types of compulsory health insurance (Chapter 8) would not be a large one.

Regardless of the ultimate outcome, however, many of these proposals could be extremely useful as devices for improving existing insurance coverage and strengthening the private sector against continuing default to public programs.

Public Financing Programs

The United States has differed from most other advanced nations in the almost total absence of public health insurance. Prior to enactment of Medicare in 1965, the only exceptions were the medical aspects of workmen's compensation and the little-known hospitalization provisions of the New York and California temporary disability laws. (The Federal Employees Program and similar programs, operated exclusively for their own employees by several state and local governments, are not usually considered public health insurance.) Despite this fact, we have followed the worldwide trend toward ever greater government participation in the financing of medical care. As early as 1960, it was estimated that the federal government alone had potential responsibility to furnish all or part of the medical care for some 31 million Americans.[17]

For years, the government share of total health care expenditures averaged about one-fourth, with the state and local portion just a little larger than the federal. This was the situation throughout the early 1960s. Starting in 1966, however, the first year of Medicare, the public share began to rise and so did the federal share vis-à-vis the state and local shares. By 1968, the public sector accounted for 37 percent of the total.[18] Estimates for 1970 place the government share at 40 percent or more, with the federal portion at about 30 percent. The government sector is now growing by leaps and bounds—even in the absence of a general health insurance program—and despite the Nixon Administration's efforts to restrain federal expenditures, Congress' decisive override of the unpopular Hill-Burton veto illustrates the point.

Table 5, next page, indicates the major public programs, with expenditures broken down by type of expenditure and by level of government support for 1968. Medicare was by far the largest, costing $6 billion. Other programs costing more than

Table 5: Public Health Care Programs: Expenditures for Services and Supplies, by Program, Type of Expenditure, and Source of Funds, 1968 (Amounts in Millions)

Program and source of funds	Total	Hospital care	Physicians' services	Dentists' services	Other professional services	Drugs and drug sundries	Eyeglasses and appliances	Nursing home care	Government public health activities	Other health services	Administration
Total	$18,719.7	$10,495.5	$2,512.4	$238.2	$151.2	$298.6	$47.3	$1,622.3	$969.0	$2,089.2	$296.0
Health insurance for the aged	5,978.9	3,844.8	1,386.4	—	64.9	—	—	351.0	—	50.1	281.7
Temporary disability insurance (medical benefits)	55.3	41.0	12.8	—	.7	.4	.4	—	—	—	—
Workmen's compensation (medical benefits)	807.5	282.6	468.4	—	24.2	16.2	16.2	—	—	—	—
Public assistance (vendor medical payments)	4,026.5	1,520.5	460.2	225.9	36.2	270.9	—	1,234.4	—	278.3	—
General hospital and medical care	2,961.1	2,936.5	4.3	.7	.8	.8	—	—	—	18.0	—
Defense Department hospital and medical care (including military dependents)	1,707.2	639.7	79.5	—	—	—	—	—	—	988.0	—
Maternal and child health services	359.6	53.2	31.2	8.0	24.4	7.6	9.7	—	—	223.2	2.2
School health	197.2	—	—	—	—	—	—	—	—	197.2	—
Other public health activities	969.0	—	—	—	—	—	—	—	969.0	—	—
Veterans' hospital and medical care	1,425.1	1,133.6	11.2	3.6	—	2.7	9.6	36.9	—	215.4	12.1
Medical vocational rehabilitation	113.3	43.6	58.4	—	—	—	11.4	—	—	—	—
Office of Economic Opportunity	119.0	—	—	—	—	—	—	—	—	119.0	—

Federal	12,175.1	6,606.8	1,779.1	121.3	103.8	143.2	24.6	996.5	488.7	1,614.9	296.0
Health insurance for the aged	5,978.9	3,844.8	1,386.4	—	64.9	—	—	351.0	—	50.1	281.7
Workmen's compensation (medical benefits)	16.2	10.4	4.0	—	1.0	.3	.3	—	—	—	—
Public assistance (vendor medical payments)	1,985.1	749.6	226.9	111.4	17.8	133.6	—	608.6	—	137.2	—
General hospital and medical care	193.6	169.0	4.3	.7	.8	.8	—	—	—	18.0	—
Defense Department hospital and medical care (including military dependents)	1,707.2	639.7	79.5	—	—	—	—	—	—	988.0	—
Maternal and child health services	176.3	27.0	23.0	5.6	19.3	5.8	6.2	—	—	87.2	2.2
Other public health activities	488.7	—	—	—	—	—	—	—	488.7	—	—
Veterans' hospital and medical care	1,425.1	1,133.6	11.2	3.6	—	2.7	9.6	36.9	—	215.4	12.1
Medical vocational rehabilitation	85.0	32.7	43.8	—	—	—	8.5	—	—	—	—
Office of Economic Opportunity	119.0	—	—	—	—	—	—	—	—	119.0	—
State and local	6,544.6	3,888.7	733.4	117.0	47.5	155.3	22.5	625.8	480.2	474.2	—
Temporary disability insurance	55.3	41.0	12.8	—	.7	.4	.4	—	—	—	—
Workmen's compensation (medical benefits)	791.4	272.2	464.4	—	23.3	15.8	15.8	—	—	—	—
Public assistance (vendor medical payments)	2,041.4	770.9	233.3	114.5	18.4	137.3	—	625.8	—	141.1	—
General hospital and medical care	2,767.5	2,767.5	—	—	—	—	—	—	—	—	—
Maternal and child health services	183.3	26.2	8.3	2.5	5.1	1.8	3.5	—	—	135.9	—
School health	197.2	—	—	—	—	—	—	—	—	197.2	—
Other public health activities	480.2	—	—	—	—	—	—	—	480.2	—	—
Medical vocational rehabilitation	28.3	10.9	14.6	—	—	—	2.8	—	—	—	—

Source: Rice, D. P., and Cooper, B. S., National health expenditures, 1929-68, *Soc. Secur. Bull.*, Jan. 1970, p. 9.

a billion dollars that year were medical assistance—mostly Medicaid—$4 billion ($2 billion federal, $2 billion state and local), the Department of Defense, $1.7 billion, and the Veterans Administration programs, $1.4 billion. Nearly $3 billion went for general hospital and medical care, mostly through state and local governments. The third largest category in the state and local column was workmen's compensation, whose medical benefits cost about $800 million in 1968.

The health programs of the Office of Economic Opportunity (OEO), while relatively modest in cost by federal budgetary standards ($119 million in 1968), have attracted widespread attention by their emphasis on the innovative concept of the neighborhood health center (Chapter 7). Forty-nine of these centers are reported to have been funded, in most of the major urban ghettos and a few rural poverty areas as well.

Space prohibits discussion of all these diverse, generally useful but largely uncoordinated, programs. Following are brief summaries of two of the most important—Medicare and Medicaid.

Medicare: Popular and Expensive

Medicare—health insurance for the aged provided under Title 18 of the Social Security Act of 1965—was the product of 20 years of public debate and controversy. Bitterly opposed by the American Medical Association, feared by many as a threat to the quality of care, especially the doctor-patient relationship, it went into effect July 1, 1966, in a provider climate that varied from outright hostility to resigned acquiescence.[19]

Four years later, Medicare is a fully accepted part of the health care scene, generally popular with providers and beneficiaries alike, and often cited by previously hostile groups as a bulwark against more "radical" programs such as Medicaid.[20]

There is good reason for this general popularity. On the consumer side, four distinct pluses must be listed: almost universal coverage of the elderly, far better benefits than any existing private health insurance available to this age group, some important improvements in the overall quality of care available to them, and relatively small costs to the aged themselves.

As of mid-1970, virtually all those 65 and over, nearly 20 million, were protected by hospital insurance under Part A, which also includes posthospital extended care and home health benefits. Approximately 95 percent, over 19 million, were also voluntarily enrolled in Part B, the medical insurance plan which also includes hospital outpatient services, home health care, physical therapy, diagnostic x-rays, and so forth. (Over 90 percent of Part B payments goes for doctors' bills, however.)[21]

As to benefit coverage, it is estimated that Medicare payments cover about half of the total health care expenditures of the elderly. For hospital and physician bills, the proportion is about three-fifths. These figures may be compared with private health insurance's record of only 36 percent for its beneficiaries (Table 3). However, this comparison does not do justice to the Medicare achievement, since it is generally acknowledged that the elderly have about two and one-half times the medical needs and costs of the general population. It was the inability of the voluntary sector to provide meaningful protection for this group that led to enactment of Medicare in the first place.

Qualitative improvements have been most evident in the area of extended care and home health services, which barely existed prior to Medicare. The quality of care available in many small hospitals, not previously inspected by the Joint Commission on Accreditation of Hospitals, has also been raised. Indeed, some hospital authorities say that the *overall* quality of hospital care has been improved, thanks partly to better financing for a group that formerly was largely indigent or medically indigent and partly to the gradual educational influence of the Medicare-required utilization review machinery. For example, Dr. John Knowles says:

> In the last two years there have been much sharper controls in our hospital than there have been in the last 160 years. . . . The utilization review committee is not only looking at the proper utilization of high-cost facilities, but is looking at the quality of patient care. . . . I can give you one example after another where bad utilization has been corrected and where quality has been improved.[22]

Finally, as to costs, Part A is financed entirely through an addition to social security taxes, paid by or on behalf of the beneficiary while he is still working. Part B is financed jointly by the covered individual, after he reaches 65, and by the federal government through general tax funds. Both parts have cost far more than originally anticipated and the impact on Medicare financing has been serious (see below). Part B contributions have had to be raised twice from the original $3.00 a month, on each party, to $5.30, effective July 1970. The hospital deductible under Part A has also been raised twice, from the original $40 to $52. In January 1971, it will go to $60. This has also resulted in a rise in the coinsurance which the patient must pay after he has been hospitalized 59 days, and in the deductible and coinsurance applicable to extended care. All of these are automatically linked to the hospital deductible.

The Part A tax on employer and employee, originally set at 0.35 percent of taxable payroll, with a limit of $6600 a year, has also been raised to 0.6 percent of $7800. It will have to be raised again, probably in 1971 (see below). Nevertheless, so far as the elderly individual is directly affected, Medicare is still a terrific bargain, primarily because the most expensive portion (Part A) is paid for by the small payroll tax, currently a maximum of $47 a year. This near-miracle of financing is made possible, of course, by means of what Winston Churchill once called "the magic of averages"—the tremendous population spread, the compulsory tax paid by the wage earner while he is working (before retirement), and the matching provisions, by employers under Part A and by the government under Part B.

On the provider side, the certainty of payment for millions of patients, previously considered "charity cases" or, at best, part payers, and the generous payment formulas—"reasonable costs" to facilities, "reasonable charges" to practitioners—have meant a substantial improvement in income for doctors, hospitals, nursing homes, and virtually every category of health care personnel and facility with any contact with the aged. It has also enabled many of them to improve the quality of their services.

Finally, the exceptionally competent administrative leadership provided by the Social Security Administration and the lengths to which SSA went to avoid disturbing preexisting institutional relationships, to involve the maximum feasible number of nongovernmental units in administration, and to permit virtually complete free choice to all beneficiaries, have all contributed to the program's general popularity.

So much for Medicare's pluses. They are impressive indeed. The minuses can almost be summed up in a single word—"cost." In the sober words of the Senate Committee on Finance Staff Study,

> The Medicare and Medicaid programs are in serious financial trouble. The two programs are also adversely affecting health care costs and financing for the general population.[23]

In three and one half years, from mid-1966 to the end of 1969, Medicare paid out more than $8.5 billion in benefits. Although its financing was established on what Congress considered to be conservative and safe actuarial assumptions, by 1970 the cost of both parts has turned out to be nearly twice as high as these assumptions. For example, the 1970 cost estimate made in 1965 for Part A was $3.1 billion; the revised estimate as of early 1970 was $5.8 billion. The federal share of Part B costs has increased from $623 million in FY 1967 to an estimated $1245 in FY 1971. The beneficiaries' share has, of course, gone up an equal amount.[24]

As already noted, taxes, contributions, coinsurance, and deductibles have had to be repeatedly raised. The Part A tax alone was raised 25 percent a little more than a year after the program started. Following recommendations of the Administration and the Ways and Means Committee, the House of Representatives voted, in May 1970, to raise the tax still further, to 1.0 percent of $9000, starting in 1971. Without such an increase the Hospital Insurance Trust Fund would be exhausted by 1973.

Medicare's financial crisis is, for the most part, the price of all the good things that have been achieved, not least the freedom of choice enjoyed by patients and the financial freedom enjoyed by most providers. As indicated, the price of Medicare coverage to individuals is still reasonable. But there are many aspects to the unexpected and unprecedented cost rise that cause grave concern. Among these are the ultimate effect on the United States economy of constantly rising regressive payroll taxes, of which the Part A tax is still only a small portion but the most rapidly rising and unpredictable portion; the possibility of re-creating a financial barrier to health care on the part of many of the elderly as the Part A deductible and coinsurance and the Part B contribution rate go up; and, perhaps most serious of all, the impact of rising Medicare (and Medicaid) prices and costs on the health care economy as a whole.

There is no question but that the remarkable inflation in health care costs that has occurred since 1965 is closely related to Medicare. Moreover, the inflation is now beginning to affect not only the price but the quality and accessibility of care for the general population.

Space prohibits full analysis of Medicare's contribution to this inflation. The subject has been dealt with extensively elsewhere, most recently in the Senate

Finance Committee study just cited. Suffice it to say that it involves both price and use of all types of services. With respect to hospitals, price is the primary culprit although there has been some rise in the average length of stay of Medicare beneficiaries. As to extended care and home health programs, both price and use have exceeded expectations. With respect to physicians' services, this is also true. Some fraud has also been revealed and widely publicized. This is less the result of any widespread dishonesty among providers or administrative laxity than of a more basic problem—maintenance of what SSA calls "program integrity" under a law that is virtually open-ended with respect to the use of physicians' services and all prices.

The Beginning of Controls

Although increasingly concerned about the cost situation, the Social Security Administration was largely helpless under the original legislation. And almost everyone was reluctant to suggest major statutory amendments, partly because the whole program was still so new, partly because it was generally felt that, on balance, Medicare was doing exceptionally well, and partly because no one was sure just what to do. In a sellers' market, even the nation's largest consumer of health care services, the federal government, was at a considerable disadvantage, short of coercive tactics which it was unwilling to use.

The first serious sign of retrenchment came in the spring of 1969 when HEW Secretary Finch, speaking for the new Administration, announced cancellation, effective July 1969, of the 2 percent "plus factor" in the Medicare hospital reimbursement formula, a relatively small but long-controversial item designed to compensate for a number of alleged shortcomings in the Medicare hospital-reimbursement formula, especially the hospital's concern over lack of adequate new capital for construction and expansion.[25]

By 1969 it was clear not only that the actuarial assumptions, tax, and contribution rates would have to be drastically revised upward, but that some way must be found to begin to discipline the "blank check" payment formulas. The Administration's principal answer to the latter was a series of legislative recommendations, known as the Cost Effectiveness Amendments of 1969. In the spring of 1970, these proposals were slightly revised, considered by the House Ways and Means Committee and, for the most part, incorporated into its omnibus Social Security Amendments of 1970—H.R.17550—reported out favorably by the Committee and adopted by the House in May.

Criticism of Medicare has been consistently harsher in the Senate Finance Committee than in the House Ways and Means Committee, as exemplified by the Senate Committee's 1969 hearings[26] and its 1970 staff report.[27] In practice, however, the Ways and Means leadership has generally prevailed in legislation.

With respect to Medicare, the following are among the major provisions of H.R.17550 (several apply equally to Medicaid):

1. The Secretary of Health, Education, and Welfare would be "required" to develop experiments and demonstrations designed to test various methods of paying providers on a "prospective" rather than "retrospective" basis. This

is the latest in a series of efforts to get away from full-cost reimbursement without going all the way to "charges."

2. The Secretary would be authorized to establish limits to "reasonable costs" based on comparisons of the cost of covered services by various classes of providers in the same geographic area. This is probably the beginning of a move toward gradations of hospitals and other facilities and graded payment rates.

3. "Reasonable charges" for physician fees would be limited, for fiscal year 1971, to the 75th percentile of actual charges in a given locality during calendar year 1969—the HEW formula devised for Medicaid payments in 1969 (see below). Thereafter, fees could be raised only in accordance with an authorized index related to the cost of living, cost of production of medical services, and other professional and managerial earnings.

4. Provider institutions would be required to have a written plan reflecting an operating budget and a capital expenditures budget.

5. The Secretary would be authorized to withhold or reduce reimbursement to providers for depreciation, interest, and other expenses related to capital expenditures over $100,000 where such expenditure is not consistent with state and regional planning agency plans.

6. Medicare would no longer pay for the services of teaching physicians unless other insured or self-pay patients were also charged for such services.

7. The Secretary would be authorized to terminate payment to any provider found guilty of fraud or other program abuses.

Perhaps the most innovative of the H.R.17550 proposals is one designed to stimulate development of health maintenance organizations (HMOs)—prepaid group practice or other capitation plans. Under this proposal, Medicare beneficiaries living in an area served by Kaiser, or any other organization which could supply both hospital and physician services, would have the option of receiving their services from such an organization rather than, as is more common, from individual doctors and hospitals. The HMO would receive its Medicare payment not in the form of reimbursement for physician visits or hospital stays, but in the form of a prospective, capitation payment, determined for each organization on an annual basis. The HMO premium could not exceed 95 percent of the cost of Parts A and B coverage for Medicare beneficiaries in the same area who were not enrolled in the HMO.

Shortly after House adoption of H.R.17550 the Secretary's Task Force on Medicaid and Related Programs (McNerney Committee) issued its long-awaited report.[28] Few of the recommendations dealt with Medicare, but two are important. One reiterated a long-standing and sensible SSA recommendation that the permanently and totally disabled social security beneficiaries—the number would be approximately 1.6 million or 2.5 depending on whether only the disabled workers were covered or their dependents were included—be brought into the program. Another urged consolidation of Parts A and B. This measure, recommended by this author as early as 1967,[29] would probably do more to help restructure and rationalize the United States health care delivery system—both organizationally and financially—than any other single reform that could be enacted in the immediate future. The HMO option represents a definite, albeit limited, step in this direction.[30]

Even before the new controls become law, SSA has begun to tighten existing administrative regulations. For example, it is now estimated that 30 percent of all bills submitted by physicians under Part B are reduced, and 8 percent are denied. The average cut is 6 percent, compared with 5.2 percent in 1969 and 2.6 percent in 1967.[31]

Medicaid: Expensive and Unpopular

Medicaid—the public assistance medical care program provided under Title 19 of the Social Security Act of 1965—differs from Medicare in almost every essential aspect. Medicare is a federal insurance program, paid for, on an actuarially determined basis, by the prospective beneficiaries and their employers, financed through special trust funds, with nationally uniform benefits, and entitlement as a matter of right, regardless of personal need. Medicaid is a series of separate state welfare programs—52 as of mid-1970[32]—paid for out of general taxes, on the basis of annual appropriations from the federal and state governments, with some federal benefit and eligibility standards but wide regional and state variations, and entitlement based on a state-administered means test. All three key variables in the Medicaid formula—the means test or income limits, benefit standards, and available funds—are subject to frequent change in accordance with economic and political pressures.

In most states, the Medicaid program is only two or three years old; in some less than a year. Definitive evaluation is thus even more difficult than in the case of Medicare. Nevertheless, certain trends are virtually inherent in the nature of the program. Moreover, the growing national crisis in health care financing and Medicaid's far reaching implications, political as well as economic, are such that the public, including providers as well as consumers, is refusing to wait for even a normal period of trial and error. Two highly placed and highly critical official critiques have already appeared—the report of the Secretary's Task Force on Medicaid and Related Programs, headed by Walter J. McNerney, President, Blue Cross Association, and the report, *Medicare and Medicaid,* prepared by the staff of the Senate Committee on Finance.[33]

Criticism has tended to focus on problems of costs and eligibility. The report of the Secretary's Task Force on Medicaid and Related Programs, for example, states at the outset:

> The promise of Medicaid that some care, at least, would be available to all who needed it has vanished into the obscurity of state determinations of eligibility and the parsimony of state determinations of solvency. How completely the promise vanished is suggested by the Task Force estimate that only about one-third of the 30-40 million indigent and medically indigent who could potentially be covered by Title XIX will, in fact, receive services. That the cost of covering less than one-third

has exceeded earlier estimates of the cost of covering the whole medically deprived population is due to a combination of factors, including inflation. It also suggests how badly the expenditures have been controlled, or how badly the program costs were estimated, or both.

In this author's view, the first part of this criticism is too harsh on the states. Title 19 eligibility standards require inclusion of all persons receiving or eligible to receive money payments under the four categorical public assistance programs— Aid to the Aged, to the Permanently and Totally Disabled, to the Blind, and to Families of Dependent Children (AFDC). Federal matching funds for Title 19 vary from 50 to 83 percent depending on a state's per capita income. The states were also encouraged to include the "medically indigent," persons not on welfare but with incomes so low that they cannot meet their medical expenses, and all children under 21 who need medical care but cannot afford it.

The definition of "medical indigence" was originally left to the states. But after New York and California had provided comparatively liberal income limits, Congress, in the 1967 Amendments to the Social Security Act, set the upper limit at one and one-third times the state's AFDC limit. This resulted in eliminating many of the medically indigent from Medicaid, especially in New York. The number of potential eligibles was also restricted by limiting the number of children under 21 who may be put on AFDC to the same proportion of all children in the state under 21 who were on AFDC Jan. 1, 1968. Additional pressure against a liberal definition of "medical indigence" comes from the fact that federal matching funds are available for only certain very limited categories of the medically indigent.

In mid-1970, slightly more than half the state programs included the latter. Wide variations exist in the eligibility limits. Under present regulations, the family income could range from a maximum of $5000 per year for a family of four in New York down to $2700 in Utah and $2600 in Puerto Rico.

By the Task Force's own estimate, some 10 million received Medicaid benefits in 1969. This may be compared with 11 million receiving cash payments under public assistance (page 18) and is 42 percent of the 24 million estimated "poor" in that year (page 17). So far as covering the very poor, those on relief, Medicaid appears to be hitting the target rather well. On the other hand, if not only the "poor" but the "near poor"—another 10 to 15 million— or all the "medically indigent"—a figure literally impossible to calculate—are included, obviously it is a much less impressive performance. But is it realistic now, or was it in 1965, to expect this program—part and parcel of our welfare-relief system—to reach all the nation's medically indigent? What logical cutoff point is there? Was it really the intention of Congress in 1965 that Medicaid should make "some care at least available to all who needed it?"

With respect to benefits, Congress has also been ambiguous. Originally, Title 19 required the states to provide all beneficiaries with at least five basic services— hospital inpatient and outpatient care, physicians' services, laboratory, and x-ray, and, for those over 21, skilled nursing home care. Fourteen other services were also eligible for federal matching. Since the 1967 Amendments, however, the states are no longer required to provide the five basic services to any but the categorically needy. For the medically needy they may substitute any 7 of the 14 others.

It should also be noted that there have never been federal standards with respect to the amount of service to be provided under the various categories—for example, the number of days of hospital care, number of physician visits, etc.

According to the original 1965 concept, it was hoped that the various categories of service would be added by the states, year by year, until they achieved the 1975 statutory goal—comprehensive health care for all who met the eligibility requirements. In 1967, however, the date was deferred to 1977, and if H.R.17550 is passed the statutory goal would be eliminated completely.

Aside from Congressional intent, is it wiser to make "some care"—which might mean as little as three days of hospitalization per year and three doctors' visits—available to all, as implied in the McNerney Task Force criticism, or to use the same limited resources to provide more meaningful benefits to a smaller number, even if that smaller number were limited to those actually on welfare? Finally, is it fair to lay all the blame for Medicaid's eligibility and benefit shortcomings on state "parsimony" and "obscurity" in view of the experience in New York and California?

With respect to costs, the critics appear to be on much firmer ground. As indicated in the Task Force quotation, the blame has to be assigned to numerous factors, including the general inflation. But the primary causes of the cost crisis are the unrealistic estimates with which the program started and the total lack of any cost controls. Viewed in relation to total national expenditures for health, or even the federal portion, Medicaid expenditures—estimated to be about $5.5 billion in FY 1970, about half federal—do not appear to be of crisis proportions. The $4 billion spent for this purpose in 1968 constituted only 7 percent of national health care expenditures for that year and 22 percent of public expenditures (Table 5).

In terms of state and local government financing, however, the Medicaid crisis is real indeed. Predictably, Medicaid has become a political football in New York and many other states. In the spring of 1969, New York and the Department of Health, Education, and Welfare moved almost simultaneously to cut back. The New York Legislature established a freeze on Medicaid payments to hospitals until the end of the year and then called for a ceiling on payments to be determined by the State Department of Health in place of the existing open-ended Medicare formula. But, also predictably, many hospitals were so badly hurt by this freeze, especially in view of the rapidly rising pay scales in the newly unionized institutions, that the Governor had to find emergency funds of various sorts to keep them afloat. The new payment ceiling also turns out to be reasonably flexible—necessarily so, if a dozen or more hospitals were not to go out of business. In due course, the Medicaid freeze was also declared unconstitutional by a federal court.

Effective July 1, 1969, HEW also announced a partial ceiling on the fees of physicians and other practitioners serving Medicaid patients. Arrived at by a special task force of providers and consumers, the formula was quite flexible, keyed to the 75th percentile of prevailing community fees, with provision for annual increases based on the BLS index of all services less medical care. Few doctors were hurt by this formula. It hardly deserved the title of a "ceiling," much less a "freeze." Nevertheless, it was significant as marking the beginning of the end of federal tolerance for completely uncontrolled fees. About the same time, the Secretary of

HEW also established the Task Force on Medicaid and Related Programs (McNerney) with instructions to review the whole picture of health care financing.

What Future for This Program?

The highly critical tone of the Task Force's report has already been noted. Its numerous recommendations deal with virtually all aspects of the health care picture from details of Title 19 state administration to reorganization of the Department of HEW, national health insurance, and even comprehensive health planning. Following are a few of the major items, dealing specifically with Medicaid:

1. Medicaid should be converted to a program "with a uniform minimum level of health benefits financed 100 percent by federal funds, with a further federal matching with states for certain types of supplementary benefits and for individuals not covered under the minimum plan."

2. Both the basic federal benefit and the supplementation should be designed to provide incentives for improved organization and delivery of services. Individual beneficiaries should be given the option to select a group practice prepayment plan.

3. "The commitment to provide comprehensive care to substantially all the needy and the medically needy should be reaffirmed." Priorities should be established now to extend coverage to additional groups—such as those who would be eligible under the Administration's proposed new Family Assistance Plan—until, as a minimum, all persons at or below the poverty level are eligible at least for the "federal benefit package." The income limit on federal participation in current medical indigency programs should be abolished.

4. With respect to immediate administrative reforms, all states should be required to simplify methods of determining eligibility, to certify eligible recipients for at least three months, and to explore the possibility of "conditional or prospective certification of the group of people with excess income to be applied to medical needs before they are eligible."

One recommendation provides that "under demonstration programs, the Social and Rehabilitation Service should help to promote availability of comprehensive health care for *all residents* in a given geographical area, combining funds from Title 19 with other sources of financing" (italics supplied).

By contrast with the wide-ranging, rather diffuse, Task Force report, the report of the Senate Committee on Finance staff is concerned exclusively with Medicare and Medicaid and its recommendations are directed solely at fiscal reform of the two programs. Among its specific proposals are the following:

1. States should be free to define "reasonable costs" as the basis of Medicaid reimbursement of hospitals in terms other than the Medicare formula, and Congressional intent on this point should be clarified.

2. Fee schedules for payment of practitioners should be required.

3. Prior professional approval of elective procedures and expensive courses of treatment should be required.

4. "Doctor shopping" by recipients should be outlawed by requiring the designation of a "primary physician."

5. States should be required to provide recipients with statements outlining payments made in their behalf.

6. Reasonable cost-sharing by the medically indigent should be permitted.

7. Vendor payments to independent collection and discount agencies should be prohibited.

8. HEW and the individual states should be required to establish special fraud and abuse units.

9. The Federal Medical Assistance Advisory Council and the Medicare Health Benefits Advisory Council should be combined "to facilitate coordination and communication in the two principal federal health care financing programs."

10. Provision for the reporting of medical payments to the Internal Revenue Service should be strengthened.

In one sense these two very different documents are complementary. The Task Force has chosen to emphasize the whole broad problem of health care delivery in the United States, and views the Medicaid crisis as only one example of the broader crisis. Its recommendations appear directed as much toward easing the transition from Medicaid to some general health care program for the entire population as to making the existing program viable. The Senate report is just the opposite. It is directed exclusively toward trying to make Medicaid work, principally by building in some effective cost controls.

It is questionable, however, whether both of these broad aims can be carried out simultaneously. Is it possible to reform and revitalize a program at the same time that we are seeking to supersede it? For thousands of federal and state employees around the country who have the responsibility for making Medicaid work this is not an academic question. Their morale and their sense of purpose are at stake. This is not the only area of modern life where one has to live with ambiguity. But at least we should recognize the ambiguity and seek to resolve the contradiction as promptly as possible.

The "Medicaid crisis" is incredibly involved. Aside from the general problems of inflation and inadequate administrative controls, which it shares with Medicare and private health insurance, the Medicaid crisis is part of the general "welfare crisis" and the "crisis in race relations." As a welfare program, paid for out of general taxes, it shares the stigma accorded by most middle-class Americans to welfare programs, especially when they appear inordinately expensive. Rejecting such limited cost controls as are present in an insurance program such as Medicare, where benefits and eligibility must be actuarially related to revenue, the Medicaid program is subject to constant pressures for both too rapid liberalization and politically explosive retrenchments.

Relying on an unadministrable means test to determine eligibility, it provides virtually an open invitation to fraud on the part of borderline consumers. As a program serving a large number of blacks, especially in northern urban areas, it is subject to the same sort of backlash resentment from low-income whites that has plagued most recent efforts to upgrade Negro social services and opportunities. It is also part of the general crisis of state and local government financing and administration. These levels of government were, for the most part, in no position to assume even half the burden of Medicaid costs. At the same time they were unprepared administratively to exercise effective cost or quality controls.

Medicaid has done some good. It has brought "mainstream" medical care— good, bad, and indifferent as it is—for the first time to several millions. It has helped to relieve many doctors, hospitals, and other providers of most of the burden of caring for the indigent and is reported to have slowed the exodus of doctors from poverty areas. However, it seems clear that the program is too unstable financially and politically, and too unwieldy administratively, to continue for any long period of time in its present form. In view of these weaknesses, the proposal that it be enlarged to take in more and more of the population seems unwise.

At the same time, it serves little purpose simply to say that it should be abolished in favor of national health insurance. The need for Medicaid could be greatly reduced through such a program, or even through improvement of Medicare and private health insurance—the most urgent next steps. It is most unlikely, however, that any insurance scheme that could be passed in the foreseeable future would be comprehensive enough to permit total abolition of Medicaid, at least for a number of years. Thus, ways must be found to strengthen the residual program. Perhaps the first order of business should be to recognize that it is, and should remain, a residual program, and to seek to do the best possible job on this basis.

The Accelerating Drift to Government Financing

Summarizing the major developments with respect to financing health care, it is obvious that the constant and accelerating rise in health care costs has been accompanied by a dramatic shift in the financing of such care from direct patient payments to third-party payments and from private third parties to the government. A recent Social Security Administration study reports that as early as FY 1968, public funds were providing nearly 90 percent of all hospital expenditures for the aged and about one-third for those under 65.[34] This means that government already accounts for over half of all hospital income.

The rise in the share of total United States health care expenditures to a 1970 estimated high of 40 percent has been noted (page 55). Even in the more restricted area of personal health care expenditures, the same trend is unmistakable. Table 6, opposite, shows the changing ratios for such expenditures from 1950 through 1968. During this period, out-of-pocket payments fell from 65 percent of the total to 41 percent. The portion paid through private health insurance rose from 9 percent to 25 percent in 1965 and then fell to 23 percent in 1968. The government share remained fairly steady, below 25 percent, until 1967, when it rose to 33 percent, reflecting the impact of Medicare and Medicaid. A year later it had reached 35 percent.

Table 6: Personal Health Care Expenditures: Amount and Percent Met by Third Parties, Selected Years 1950-68
(Amounts in Millions)

| Year | Personal health care expendi-tures* | Direct payments | | Third-party payments | | | | | | | |
| | | | | Total | | Private health insurance | | Government | | Philanthropy and others | |
		Amount	Percent	Amount	Percent	Amount	Percent	Amount	Percent	Amount	Percent
1950.........	$11,109	$ 7,209	64.9	$ 3,900	35.1	$ 992	8.9	$ 2,588	23.3	$320	2.9
1955.........	15,933	9,271	58.2	6,662	41.8	2,536	15.9	3,705	23.3	421	2.6
1960.........	23,758	13,068	55.0	10,690	45.0	4,996	21.0	5,157	21.7	537	2.3
1965.........	34,942	18,171	52.0	16,771	48.0	8,729	25.0	7,345	21.0	697	2.0
1966.........	38,794	19,374	49.9	19,420	50.1	9,142	23.6	÷ 9,534	24.6	744	1.9
1967.........	44,202	19,342	43.8	24,860	56.2	9,545	21.6	†14,550	32.9	765	1.7
1968.........	49,895	20,348	40.8	29,550	59.2	11,310	22.7	†17,455	35.0	785	1.6

*All expenditures for health services and supplies other than (a) expenses for prepayment and administration, (b) government public activities, and (c) expenditures of private voluntary agencies for other health services.

†Includes benefit payments under health insurance for the aged (Medicare).

Source: Rice, D. P., and Cooper, B. S., National health expenditures, 1929-68, Soc. Secur. Bull., Jan. 1970, p. 17.

If current trends continue, the public share will rise to 50 percent or more in a few years. Anything more than half would mark the end of our predominantly private medical care economy and the beginning of a whole new government-dominated ball game. This is true despite the fact that government in the United States has been demonstrably reluctant to exercise real leadership, let alone domination, with respect to patient care institutions. Regardless of such reluctance, the realities of fiscal accountability in a period of rapid inflation would inevitably force the public agencies to adopt far-reaching controls.

The primary cause for the shift to government financing has not been inefficiency on the part of the carriers or any *a priori* preference for government financing on the part of consumers. The primary cause has been the unabating rise in medical care costs which, in turn, derives primarily from the increasing imbalance between supply and demand. While money has been literally poured into demand, the steps taken to increase supply or its effectiveness have generally been too little and too late.

* * *

Here, then, is Paradox Number Four: Thanks to the tremendous recent expansion of both public and private financing programs, the financial barrier to health care has been substantially reduced for most Americans. The vast majority are now protected, to a greater or lesser degree, by one or more such programs. The providers have benefited at least as much. Many exciting innovations have emerged. Yet shortcomings in the programs, especially Medicaid, the continuing gaps and duplications and, above all, the ever-rising provider costs—now reaching critical dimensions—have meant inability to provide comprehensive coverage and continuing dissatisfaction on the part of both providers and consumers. In some states and communities where programs have had to be cut back, the political repercussions, combined with other explosive factors in the American city, have contributed to a crisis situation in the strictest meaning of the term.

NOTES

1. For the large regional and state variation in per capita expenditures, see, Reed, L. S. and Carr, W., Per capita expenditures for hospital care, the services of physicians and dentists, and private health insurance, by region and state, 1966. U.S. Department of Health, Education, and Welfare, Social Security Administration, *Research and Stat. Note 13*, Aug. 1, 1969.

2. For the most exhaustive recent analysis of health care expenditures, see, Klarman, H. E., Rice, D. P., Cooper, B. S., and Stettler, H. L., Accounting for the rise in selected medical care expenditures, 1929-69. *Amer. J. Public Health*, June 1970, pp. 1023-39. The authors show that over the four decades, prices contributed one-half the increase; population growth, one-sixth; per capita use and quality, about one-third.

3. Blue Cross of Southwest Ohio, *Perspective*, Second Quarter 1970, pp. 3-4.

4. For the historical development of health insurance and a review of major programs, carriers, and problems, as of the early 1960s, see Somers, H. M. and A. R., *Doctors, Patients, and Health Insurance* (Brookings Institution, 1961), pp. 225-27, 249-451.

5. For a brief objective report on the Kaiser Plan, see, National Advisory Commission on Health Manpower, *Report*, Vol. II, Nov. 1967, Appendix IV, pp. 197-228.

6. Health Insurance Institute, *Source Book of Health Insurance Data, 1969* (New York City), p. 11.

7. Reed, L. S., Private health insurance, 1968: enrollment, coverage, and financial experience. U.S. Department of Health, Education, and Welfare, *Soc. Secur. Bull.,* Dec. 1969, p. 19. All data in this section are from this source unless otherwise indicated.

8. Cohen, W., National health insurance: problems and prospects, Michael M. Davis Lecture, University of Chicago, 1970, pp. 3-4.

9. For a comprehensive report on one such plan, Group Health Dental Insurance of New York, see, Avnet, H. H. and Nikias, M. K., *Insured Dental Care* (New York City: Group Health Dental Insurance, Inc., 1967).

10. For a detailed survey of benefit provisions under various types of private insurance, see, Reed, L. S. and Carr, W., The benefit structure of private health insurance, 1968. Social Security Administration, Office of Research and Statistics, *Research Report No. 32,* 1970.

11. *Med. World News,* July 25, 1969, p. 26G.

12. United Mine Workers of America Welfare and Retirement Fund, *Report 1968,* p. 3. Also, Gooden, O., Office of Executive Medical Officer, Letter to author, Nov. 19, 1968.

13. Saward, E. W., The relevance of prepaid group practice to the effective delivery of health services. Reprinted by U.S. Department of Health, Education, and Welfare, Health Services and Mental Health Administration, Office of Group Practice Development.

14. See, for example, McNerney, W. J., Improving the effectiveness of health insurance and prepayment. U.S. Department of Health, Education, and Welfare, Social Security Administration, *Private Health Insurance and Medical Care,* Conference Papers, 1968, pp. 43-73.

15. See, for example, Pettengill, D. W., A program to improve the availability, acceptability, and financing of health care for all in the United States. Presented to U.S. House of Representatives, Committee on Ways and Means, Washington, D.C., Nov. 6, 1969. Also, Health Insurance Association of America, *Health Care Delivery in the 1970's:* Report, Findings, and Recommendations, Adopted by the Board of Directors, Oct. 28, 1969.

16. For discussion of FEP, its benefits, costs, and some comparisons with Medicare, see, Somers, A. R., What price comprehensive care? *Arch. Environ. Health,* July 1968, pp. 8-20. Also, periodic reports from U.S. Civil Service Commission.

17. U.S. Bureau of the Budget, The budget of the U.S. government for the FY ending June 30, 1960, *Special Analysis J.,* p. 1004.

18. Rice, D. P. and Cooper, B. S., National health expenditures, 1929-68. *Soc. Secur. Bull.* Jan. 1970, p. 4.

19. For the historical development of the Medicare legislation and discussion of the program as of the first year of operation, see, Somers, H. M. and A. R., *Medicare and the Hospitals* (Brookings Institution, 1967).

20. For example, a quarter-page ad in the *New York Times,* sponsored by the Suffolk County Medical Society, as early as June 10, 1966, opposing the New York Medicaid law, starts, "I am a doctor. . . . I will cooperate fully with the provisions of the Federal Medicare Law which provides a sensible and reasonable plan of medical care for all people over 65 . . ."

21. For detailed review of Medicare, see U.S. Department of Health, Education, and Welfare, Social Security Administration, *Operation of Medicare Program—Annual Report* (starting 1968). Also, Health Insurance Benefits Advisory Council, *Annual Report* (starting 1969). For statistical data, see *Soc. Secur. Bull.,* current operating statistics (monthly) and periodic reports from the Division of Research and Statistics.

22. Knowles, J., The physician in the decade ahead. *Hospitals, J.A.H.A.,* Jan. 1, 1970, p. 58.

23. 91st Congress, 1st Session, *Medicare and Medicaid: Problems, Issues, and Alternatives,* Report of the Staff to the Committee on Finance, U.S. Senate, 1970, p. 1.

24. *Ibid.,* pp. 3-4.

25. For the history of the "plus factor" and other components of the hospital reimbursement formula, see, Somers, *Medicare and the Hospitals, op. cit.* (Note 19), Chapter VIII.

26. 91st Congress, 1st Session, *Medicare and Medicaid,* Hearings before the Committee on Finance, U.S. Senate, July 1 and 2, 1969.

27. See Note 23, above.

28. U.S. Department of Health, Education, and Welfare, Office of the Secretary, *Recommendations of the Task Force on Medicaid and Related Programs,* 1970.

29. Somers, *Medicare and the Hospitals, op. cit.,* p. 269.

30. For the Task Force's discussion of the HMO proposal, including the recommendation that the 95 percent limitation be deleted, see, *Recommendations of the Task Force on Medicaid and Related Programs, op. cit.,* pp. 33-36.

31. *Med. Econ.* Mar. 30, 1970, p. 32.

32. Forty-eight states, District of Columbia, Puerto Rico, Virgin Islands, and Guam. Arizona and Alaska have no programs. For information on Medicaid, see, U.S. Department of Health, Education, and Welfare, Social and Rehabilitation Service, Medical Services Administration.

33. See Notes 28 and 23.

34. *Med. Econ.* Nov. 10, 1969, p. 20.

PART TWO

From Paradox to New Progress:
Goals and Guidelines

> The great social dilemma is that liberals, conservatives and reactionaries have all fallen victim to the myth that the only barrier standing between a person and good medical care is his inability to pay for it. We have adequately demonstrated by the wide extension of third-party payment mechanisms, public or private, that that is not true. There are many people, rich and poor, who essentially are not faced with the problem of payment but who cannot find the medical care. They cannot even find the doctor or the system. . . .
>
> IRVING J. LEWIS
> *New England Journal of Medicine* (October 16, 1969)

> This is the day of the iatrogenic illness, the illness caused by the medicine itself. Any government department, indeed any organization setting out to cure social ills, had better be sure it isn't creating problems as rapidly as it cures them.
>
> JOHN W. GARDNER
> *No Easy Victories* (1968)

The "massive crisis" in health care, referred to by President Nixon, July 10, 1969, is no new or sudden development. On the contrary, it has been gathering momentum over several decades and was predicted by health care authorities as far back as the early 1930s in the reports of the Committee on the Costs of Medical Care.[1]

Nor is it attributable to any one factor—physicians, hospitals, the pharmaceutical industry, third-party carriers, government, unions, or patients. In the complex scientific and demographic calculus that has led to the current crisis, key elements of which were discussed in Part One, all parties have played a role. All have contributed to the problem.

This does not imply that any of these actors are villains: The medical specialist concentrating on one small orifice or area of the body to the neglect of the whole man; the hospital seeking to meet all the complex and contradictory demands put upon it, to the neglect of rational organization and economy; the insurance carrier seeking to meet the buyers' most pressing demand for hospitalization benefits, as well as the insurance industry's traditional concept of "insurability," to the neglect of ambulatory care; the patient pleading for the latest miracle drug or miracle surgery to the neglect of routine diet and exercise; the union leader jumping on the national health insurance bandwagon as the seemingly quickest way of obtaining adequate financing for needed health services.

[1] For this and succeeding notes in this introduction, see page 78.

All are responding to the scientific and technological revolution in medicine, each in his own way, each betraying his own humanity, which by definition means a mixture of strength and weakness, good and bad.

But just as each participant has been part of the problem, so is he also part of the solution. This is a fairer statement than the VISTA motto, "If you are not part of the solution, you are part of the problem." Obviously, we are all both. Just as the far-sighted members of the Committee on the Costs of Medical Care could antici-pate, nearly 40 years ago, the now-current crisis, so is it possible to discern, on the basis of present developments, the shape of solutions, and still more problems, to come.

The four paradoxes, discussed in Chapters 1 through 4, are all part of what might be called the general paradox of progress. All creative achievement is dis-ruptive. Every partial solution promptly leads to a new set of problems. The in-creasing application of science and technology to our lives means more frequent dislocations and more violent contradictions. Conflict, so often deplored, and even temporary regression may be the inevitable handmaidens of progress. It is ironic, but should not be surprising, that widespread criticism of the health care Estab-lishment and of financing mechanisms has developed precisely at the time when such care is better and more accessible than ever before.

But such philosophical thoughts, while intellectually comforting, provide no ex-cuse for complacency or inaction. On the contrary, they suggest that the real solution to the present health care dilemma in the United States may have to be more radical than is generally realized. But "radical" does not necessarily mean more government operation. Just turning the problem over to government, because of greater ease of financing, might be the easiest, but also the laziest and in the long run most unproductive, approach to the problem. In terms of our basic ap-proach to health care, we seem to have painted ourselves into a corner, qualitatively as well as financially. If we are to get out of this corner, we must do some basic rethinking. This rethinking must involve all aspects of the health care equation—organization as well as financing, prevention and aftercare as well as diagnosis and treatment, consumer knowledge as well as provider skills, the doctor-patient rela-tionship as well as the science and technology of medicine.

A second general point has to do with the basic questions "Are we falling apart as a society?" and "Is there now, not one, but two Americas?" At first glance it is tempting to say "Yes!" The human picture that emerges from the statistics in Chapter 2 is full of glaring contrasts: large pockets of poverty amid the general affluence; a simultaneous rise in employment, earnings, and welfare rolls; higher family incomes and more broken homes.

On the one hand, there is the world of the affluent majority, attuned to the staccato rhythm of a dynamic, technologically oriented, upwardly mobile society, for whom life is far easier than it was for their grandparents or even their parents, richer not only in material goods but in broader intellectual and cultural horizons—the Americans for whom the moon shots have become a symbol of man's near-conquest of his environment.

Then, on the other hand, there is the "other America"—not only the millions of functional illiterates, black and white, trapped in urban or rural ghettos of poverty and ignorance, but the millions of homeless old people languishing in cheerless nursing homes, the millions of retarded or emotionally disturbed children, of frustrated, middle-aged businessmen and professionals who just couldn't "make it," and, perhaps saddest of all, the intelligent but embittered youthful dropouts from the affluent technological society—the Americans for whom the moon shots are a mockery, a callous diversion of national resources which, they believe, might otherwise be available to ease their lot on earth.

Despite the contrasts and even contradictions in life styles in the United States today, however, a more careful reading of the statistics suggests strongly that there is more uniformity than diversity. We are still far from homogeneity but we are tending in that direction. If poverty seems so widespread, it is at least partly because our definition of poverty is so much more generous than in the past—a generosity made possible only by the pervasive affluence and the impressive technological base upon which it rests. If the welfare rolls continue to grow, it is partly because our reaction to poverty is more humane than in the past and this again is possible only because of the technological foundation. The aged, the physically and emotionally crippled, the retarded, the youthful dropouts are visible and increasingly vocal because technological, economic, and medical progress have enabled us to keep them alive and give them a certain status in society. The black revolution is upon us not because conditions are worse than they used to be but because they are better. The blacks, too, have been caught up in the revolution of rising expectations and will no longer be mute victims of social injustice.

This point—that the current crisis is the result of progress rather than retrogression or decay—is vitally important not only as a historical fact but as a guide to problem solving in the health field as elsewhere.[2] If there really were two Americas, we would have to design and operate two health care systems. If, on the other hand, there is only one America with varying degrees of achievement of the American ideal of "life, liberty and the pursuit of happiness," then the object is to design a single system with enough flexibility—regional, financial, ethnic, and other variations—to allow for the persistent differentials, and then seek to close the gap and to raise the standards of the less-advantaged groups.

The time has come to suggest some means of resolving the four paradoxes and, in so doing, to establish some guidelines for our evolving health care system. Part One focused on the past and the present—how we got where we are. Part Two focuses on the future—how to get from where we are to where we want to be. Its aim is to help in the development of a new national health care policy appropriate to the scientific, technological, and demographic facts of life in the 1970s. It does this not by means of any theoretical formulation but by concentrating on some realistic possibilities—practical options—for corrective action. The theoretical commitments have already been made. As noted in Chapter 2, we are already committed, as a nation, "to assure comprehensive health services of high quality for every person." The challenge now is to make this commitment meaningful, to translate it into tangible goods and services and, ultimately, into longer life and better health for all Americans.

The points selected for emphasis in Chapters 5 through 8 appear especially significant in terms of both urgency and the inadequacy of current public discussion.

No effort has been made to achieve totality or complete answers. For example, millions of consumer-patients obviously require surgery and other types of acute care. Health education and health maintenance, the subjects of Chapter 5, have been emphasized in the effort to correct their long neglect, but this should not be taken as a recommendation for the opposite fallacy. Similarly, numerous important problems bearing on the organization of physician services, community health services, and financing have been omitted.

Also, needless to say, all of the points discussed in these four chapters are interrelated. But each one is so complex that it has to be thought about separately and separate action-strategies devised. The concept of comprehensive care and the idea of a total approach to the solution of health care problems are highly satisfying philosophically but, as a matter of practical necessity, the concept has to be broken down into its principal component parts and achievement of these components pursued in the usual pluralistic and pragmatic fashion typical of American social reform programs.[3]

NOTES

1. This committee of 50 distinguished citizens, under the chairmanship of Dr. Ray Lyman Wilbur, President Hoover's Secretary of the Interior and President of Stanford University, published 28 volumes on all aspects of medical care, 1927-32. The final volume, *Medical Care for the American People* (Chicago: University of Chicago Press, 1932), has become a classic.

2. For a similar approach to the diagnosis and treatment of other social problems, see, Farson, R. E., How could anything that feels so bad be so good? *Saturday Review*, Sept. 6, 1969, p. 20 ff.

3. For some earlier efforts to deal pragmatically with the problem of comprehensive care, see, Somers, A. R., What price comprehensive care? *Arch. Environ. Health*, July 1968, pp. 6-20. Also, How does comprehensive health care relate to the health care industry? *Arch. Physical Med. and Rehab.*, Oct. 1969, pp. 556-62.

Chapter 5

A NATIONAL PROGRAM OF CONSUMER HEALTH EDUCATION

The greatest potential for improving the health of the American people is not to be found in increasing the number of physicians or in forcing them into groups, or even in increasing hospital productivity, but is to be found in what people do and don't do to, and for, themselves. With so much attention given to medical care and so little to health education and individual responsibility for personal health, we run the danger of pandering to the urge to buy a quick solution to a difficult problem.

VICTOR R. FUCHS
Medical Economics (February 5, 1968)

A very substantial portion of acute illness is the accumulated end results of the individual's personal living habits. . . . Positive health is not something one human being can give to, or require of, another. In large part, its attainment must include self-directed, intelligent, continuing, personal effort. Absent that effort, the health services can only insulate the individual from the more catastrophic results of his ignorance, self-indulgence, or lack of motivation. Providers of health services must learn increasingly to work with patients rather than to do things to or for them. Until we do, our task will exceed our strengths. For that reason, I place first priority on the development, continuing updating, and pervasive distribution of teaching materials for use by parents in the home, by peer groups, and in the primary grades.

J. DOUGLAS COLMAN
Hilleboe Memorial Lecture (1970)

The nation's health strategy must now emphasize health maintenance through preventive medicine, health education, and environmental management, in addition to treatment.

Report of the 37th American Assembly (1970)

As noted in Chapter 2, many of the nation's major health problems, including automobile accidents, alcoholism, drug addiction, venereal disease, obesity, premature birth, certain cancers, and much heart disease, are primarily attributable not to shortcomings on the part of the providers of care but to ignorance or irresponsibility of the individual consumer or the community as a whole. This has always been true. But in the past, when ignorance and poor health were so often associated with poverty, there was a tendency to believe that reduction in poverty would almost automatically bring better health. The health-threatening aspects of affluence, discussed in Chapter 2, were not understood. Today, however, there is little excuse for continued blindness on this point. Findings such as

79

those reported in the Auster-Leveson-Sarachek study, that high income is positively associated with high mortality unless offset by education and medical care (page 22), make clear the absolute necessity for priority emphasis on education.

The teen-age child of wealthy parents who turns to drugs for everything from weight control, to complexion control, to constipation, to birth control, to keeping awake to study for an exam, to going to sleep after the exam is over, and to finding togetherness, peace, and happiness in an alien world, is looking for trouble just as surely as the middle-aged businessman who eats too much, drinks too much, smokes too much, takes no exercise, and spends most of his free time sitting in front of TV.

So here is one more paradox to cope with: The 10 million Americans who don't have enough to eat live side by side with 40 million others who eat too much.[1]

The Uninformed Consumer: Threat to Any Health Care System

Given our national commitment to "comprehensive health services of high quality for every person," such individuals are not only endangering their own health but building up a formidable health care bill for the nation as a whole and are a threat to the future viability of any health care system. The commitment assumes rational individual responsibility for one's own health. Without this ingredient, the commitment cannot possibly be honored.

Moreover, the community or nation that permits its air and water supplies to be poisoned, its food contaminated by harmful additives, the safety of its streets and highways threatened by drug addicts and drunken drivers, the welfare of its children undermined by too many unwanted babies, and the health of its senior citizens eroded through inactivity and a general sense of uselessness: such a community or nation makes a mockery of its professed commitment to health and safety.

The medical profession cannot be held responsible for the individual or collective irresponsibility of millions of American patient-consumers and their poor health. Indirectly, however, the profession and other providers are responsible for abdicating one of their most important roles—that of health educators. Individual doctors and a few medical societies do the best they can on this score, but the profession as a whole has been either silent or ineffective with respect to many of the major problems such as air and water pollution, cigarette smoking, overuse of drugs, birth control, automobile safety, food additives, and so forth. By failure to assume leadership on such issues doctors have not only contributed to the patients' own irresponsibility but have helped to build up the formidable demand for medical services that is now threatening the entire health care economy.

For example, a recent study of automobile accidents concluded:

> More and more physicians, as well as nonmedical specialists, are coming to the conclusion that another massive part of the highway accident epidemic is really a problem in public health and preventive medicine and that the medical profession bears a heavy share of the responsibility for its solution. Drug effects are but one of the medical factors.[2]

[1]For this and succeeding notes in this chapter, see page 85.

Even doctors and institutions that specialize in "preventive medicine," such as "executive health examinations," have all too often been so preoccupied with the mechanics of early diagnosis and the measurement of "yield" that they neglect the even more important aspect of prevention—education of the asymptomatic patient to maintain his own health. Providers as well as consumers have a large stake in the development of an effective national system of health education.

New Responsibilities for the Patient-Consumer

In recent years, new dimensions have been added to the problem. It is now necessary for the consumer to learn not only how to prevent illness, to the best of his ability, but how to help in the treatment once he is ill. Dr. Michael Crichton has underscored this point:

> It is a fact of medical life, which can be dated quite precisely in terms of origin: it began in 1923, with Banting and Best. The discovery of insulin by these workers led directly to the first chronic therapy of complexity and seriousness, where administration lay in the hands of the patient. Prior to that time, there were indeed chronic medications—such as digitalis for heart failure or colchicine for gout—but a patient taking such medications did not need to be terribly careful about it or terribly knowledgeable about his disease process. That is to say, if he took his medicines irregularly, he developed medical difficulties fairly slowly, or else he developed difficulties that were not life-threatening.

> Insulin was different. A patient had to be careful or he might die in a matter of hours. And since insulin there has come a whole range of chronic therapies that are equally complex and serious, and that require a knowledgeable, responsible patient.

> Partly in response to these demands, partly as a consequence of better education, patients are more knowledgeable about medicine than ever before. Only the most insecure and unintelligent physicians wish to keep patients from becoming even more knowledgeable.[3]

Thus, the patient must now also become a member of the health care team. Indeed, unless the professional members of that team become better organized and better oriented—both to each other and to the patient—the latter may end up, by default, as "captain" of the team, the one who has to make the choices, however uninformed, among various specialties and modalities. This is a role that most consumers surely do not want and, if the changes suggested in Chapters 6 and 7 are put into effect, it can be avoided. In any case, however, it is clear that the consumer must be prepared and educated to play an informed, responsible role in his own treatment and cure—especially in cases of chronic or mental illness.

Now it appears that the demand for consumer participation is being advanced still further. It has recently become customary for government to require a majority, or at least a substantial number, of consumers on most health care advisory boards. Third-party payers, hospitals, neighborhood health centers are all required or urged to include meaningful consumer representation. In some instances where this has not been done fast enough, self-appointed spokesmen for consumers have taken power into their own hands, going so far as to "occupy" or take over health facilities.

The move toward "consumerism," "Naderism," or "consumer participation" in health care, as in other aspects of American life, reflects many diverse factors—political and economic as well as health.

Many health care providers have resisted this trend, which they see as the "politicalization" of health care or as a threat to the quality of care. These are real dangers. Just now there is an inordinate amount of fumbling and wasted time going on in this respect. Neither the new consumer representatives nor the providers, working with them, know quite what is expected of them. But for the long run this is a promising development. It provides a good opportunity to educate key individuals who, in turn, can help to educate their fellow consumers. The union officials who have participated for some years in running their local health and welfare funds have learned something about the limits, as well as the cost, of health care and are no longer so unreasonable in their demands or expectations. The black mothers who are serving on advisory committees for neighborhood health centers are going through the same educational process.

For better or worse, however, the health care "consumer" is here to stay as part of the health care picture. Since he is ultimately footing the $64 billion bill, he is going to have some say, either directly through the provider institutions, or indirectly through government, or through both. It would appear the wiser course, from the point of view of the providers, to encourage direct participation. It would also appear the course of wisdom to do everything possible to promote effective programs in health education for all citizens, starting, as J. Douglas Colman has suggested, in the home, and continuing through school, college, and adult life.

Failures and Opportunities

The idea of health education is far from radical. Something under this name has been taught in schools of public health for many years. Many elementary and secondary schools have courses officially labeled "health education" or some synonym. However, as is generally known, they have not been successful in reaching the youngsters. For the most part, these courses have little relation to real-life problems and show no imagination. Start with a lecture on the evils of smoking, either tobacco or marijuana, and the instructor might as well give up immediately. But start with a realistic discussion of drugs, or sex, or weight problems, and a skillful instructor may be able to lay a basis for lifetime understanding of the use and abuse of drugs, nutrition, exercise, healthy marital relations, and general self-control.

The point is frequently made that education alone is inadequate, that knowledge does not necessarily lead to desirable changes of behavior. Of course this is true, but it does not follow that education is useless. The point is to relate education to personal experience, to give meaning to this experience, to help the youngster anticipate future experience, good and bad, and, above all, to avoid hypocrisy and half-truths.

Young people are frequently more concerned about illness and health than adults think they are. The enthusiasm with which college students have recently climbed on the "ecology bandwagon" may not appear entirely persuasive to some long-time critics of air and water pollution. Nevertheless, all converts, genuine or otherwise, must be welcomed.

Youthful awareness of personal health problems is far deeper than is often realized. So long as the possibility of death or maiming in a distant war, which appears to have neither purpose nor end, hangs like the sword of Damocles over most young males, it is unrealistic to expect them to get too excited over the possible ill effects of marijuana or speeding. Moreover, adults must appreciate the extent to which more or less deliberate self-abuse may be seen as a means of rebuking the older generation for the many negative aspects of the American life style—a life style in which war, violence, racial prejudice, overpopulation, and environmental pollution play such conspicuous roles.

The fact remains that the majority of young Americans, like the majority of their elders, want to be healthy and appreciate intelligent help in that direction. For example, a recent study by the American Cancer Society reports that a majority of American teen-agers oppose smoking, but environmental magnets like advertisements and the habits of parents and peers still draw about 40 percent to smoking.[4]

We desperately need a new approach to curricula, teaching materials, and teaching techniques at the elementary and secondary school levels. Obviously, this also calls for a redefinition of health education at the teacher-training level and a whole new innovative approach in the schools of public health and medicine.

Health Education for the Entire Population

The current multimillion dollar business in do-it-yourself health books, magazines, and articles, the popularity of "health" food stores and their ever-growing coterie of dedicated diet-conscious customers, the success of Weight Watchers and other "health clubs" outside the health care Establishment all testify to the widespread hunger for intelligent, informative health guidance. This attitude is probably far more widespread than the irresponsibility we have already noted, although the two are not necessarily incompatible.

The official attitude of the medical profession and of the U.S. Food and Drug Administration has generally been one of contemptuous opposition to all such "extra-Establishment" activities. Given the inability of most doctors to find time to deal with such problems, it would be far more helpful to light a few candles of effective health education than to curse the darkness.

Where such candles have been lit they have generally been well received. The work of the Planned Parenthood-World Population Association provides an outstanding example of professional leadership in tackling a difficult and profoundly serious sociohealth problem. The effectiveness of the antismoking campaign on television, sponsored primarily by the American Cancer Society and the American Heart Association, is testified to by the slight recent decline in cigarette consumption. For many years the Metropolitan Life Insurance Company did a fine job on radio with its health education messages. The AMA, Blue Cross, and Blue

Shield do some of this in some areas today, both on radio and TV. They have barely scratched the surface.

The importance of television in the continuing health education of adults and young people alike cannot be exaggerated. The negative effects are with us constantly. Even with the new antismoking ads, teen-agers are exposed to more than three times as many messages supporting smoking as assailing it.[5] Heroin and LSD are not sold on TV, but the drug habit is. Clearly there is need for some national policy, guidelines, and leadership with respect to use of television and other mass media for this purpose.

Moreover, words and actions should be made compatible. If a life insurance company undertook to back up its health messages with the requirement that every policyholder have a physical checkup once a year, the effect on those policyholders would probably be considerably greater. It wouldn't be necessary to send the results to the company. Some companies give reduced rates to nonsmokers. Why not all?

The desirability and the possibility of dietary revision for the entire population are just beginning to be seriously debated. For example, Dr. Jeremiah Stamler, Executive Director, Chicago Health Research Foundation, and a leading advocate of dietary management, estimates that a nationwide switchover to cholesterol-lowering diets could save the lives of thousands of persons each year who now die prematurely of coronary artery disease.[6] Dr. Stamler's view is opposed by equally prestigious authorities who say we do not yet have enough definitive information. The exchange is reminiscent of the early debate over fluoridation of the water supply.

It might be desirable to require all third parties, public and private, to devote one percent of their health care revenue to general health education. All schools of the health professions and all hospitals could be required to allocate a similar percentage of their budgets to the same cause.

Of course, the one individual with the greatest potential as a health educator is the doctor. He is the one who sees the patient when he is most receptive to health counsel. He is the one who is really listened to. Here is a great "teachable moment," and there is either a positive or negative educational outcome depending upon the quality of the doctor-patient relationship during the time they are together. Some doctors are making an earnest effort to incorporate patient education into their daily patient contacts. But most doctors today are too busy to take on this extra burden. And even if they had time, many lack both the inclination and the general knowledge to do the job effectively. This is the price of modern specialization. It is a high price—so high, in terms of frequently ineffective medical care as well as frequent patient dissatisfaction, that some corrective action cannot be delayed much longer. This is the subject of Chapter 6.

Some hospitals also give lip service to the concept of consumer health education. A few, such as Lankenau in Philadelphia, do something about it. In 1964 the AHA, in cooperation with the Metropolitan Life Insurance Company, sponsored an interesting conference on the subject.[7] The net results are almost zero. Most hospitals are totally unprepared for this work. However, with a little imagination, a little money, and the cooperation of the medical staff, patient education could be effectively tied to patient care (Chapter 7).

A National Council on Health Education

In order to provide a national center for interest, expertise, promotion, and evaluation in all the areas of actual or potential health education noted in this chapter, the establishment of a permanent high-level National Council on Health Education is recommended. The council would be responsible for formulation of national policy in such areas as:

- National goals with respect to health education
- Teacher training for formal health education courses
- Curricula for grade schools and colleges
- Programs for adult education
- Programs for the mass media
- Health education in hospitals and other public or publicly supported institutions
- Health education and the insurance industry
- Consumer participation in health care programs as a technique of health education

Membership should include the leadership of the medical profession, schools of health professions, hospitals, and other provider groups; business, labor, minority, and other consumer groups; third-party carriers; and government. The council should be advisory to the Secretary of Health, Education, and Welfare and organizationally sited in his office.

In the first instance, it should undertake a thorough evaluation of existing efforts in health education and develop a new package that would add up to a meaningful national program. Thereafter, it would periodically evaluate ongoing programs and reformulate policy to meet new needs. The council should be adequately funded, imaginatively staffed, including experts in audiovisual techniques, and prepared to play a leadership role vis-à-vis the health and education establishments and the mass media.

NOTES

1. The great American paradox. *Med. World News,* Nov. 28, 1969, pp. 24-33. For details with respect to both aspects of this paradox and some recommendations, see, White House Conference on Food, Nutrition, and Health (Jean Mayer, Chairman) *Report to the President,* Dec. 31, 1969.
2. Reducing highway slaughter. *Med. World News,* Oct. 24, 1969, p. 24.
3. Crichton, M., *Five Patients: The Hospital Explained* (New York: Knopf, 1970), pp. 217-18.
4. *New York Times,* Oct. 7, 1969.
5. *Ibid.*
6. Atherosclerosis: the growing national debate over serum cholesterol, lipid metabolism, genetics, and life style. *Med. World News,* Apr. 17, 1970, p. 37.
7. American Hospital Association, *Health Education in the Hospital,* 1965.

Chapter 6

REDEFINITION OF PROFESSIONAL ROLES TO ASSURE PERSONALIZED CARE

Participation of the patient in the policy-making process will be essential to the launching of a viable computer-based system that is to have hope of gaining widespread acceptance. It can be expected that the patient, as the ultimate judge of the product, will protest if the improvements structured by experts fail to satisfy community needs and to preserve individual dignity. Indeed, the most creative efforts to implement effective information systems are likely to flounder if the individual is made to feel that he is simply raw material in an impersonal medical processing plant.

WILLIAM B. SCHWARTZ, M.D.
New England Journal of Medicine (December 3, 1970)

What is the clinician? Is he a biochemist, a biophysicist, a biologist, a pathologist, a psychologist, a psychiatrist, a social scientist, a statistician? He is none of these, and at the same time, he must be something of all of them. Something akin to a chemical change must take place, a new compound, a new entity must be formed. . . . We are just beginning to understand the mysterious ingredient, the powerful therapeutic influence of the physician, of the hospital, of the clinic, of the placebo. It may well be that this mysterious ingredient has been the principal determinant of the survival of the medical profession over the centuries.

JOHN ROMANO, M.D.
Journal of Medical Education (July 1963)

Medicine still often amounts to one man asking another for help.

MICHAEL HALBERSTAM, M.D.
New York Times Magazine (November 9, 1969)

Both the need for, and the movement toward, some sort of system of health care are indisputable. Systemization is not only inevitable but desirable. It is the only way that the demand for health care can be met. Moreover, systemization and personalization are not necessarily antithetical. On the contrary, only if we fully exploit the potential of the computer, modern transportation and communications systems, and highly developed organizational relationships can we even hope to provide first-rate personal medical attention to the more than 200 million Americans to whom we have made a national commitment.

There is, however, an ever-present danger in this engineering approach, the danger that we become so enamored with the challenge of systems building or the efficiency of technological diagnosis that we forget one of the major purposes of it all—educating the patient to understand and to cope successfully with his health problems. If health planners and legislators should lose sight of the human values and relationships that are essential to realization of this goal—the satisfaction of the health professional in his work and the satisfaction of the patient with the services he is receiving—all the fine systems and the organizational designs will probably be repudiated, both by the professions and the public, even if it means going back to the obsolete nonsystem of the past.

In brief, the challenge is to create a system that will give us the best of both worlds—the world of advanced science, technology, heavy capital investment, sophisticated management, specialized personnel, and systems engineering, and also the world of individual freedom, individual responsibility, respect for privacy and human dignity, understanding of the holistic or psychosomatic nature of health and disease, and appreciation of the need of human beings for other human beings.

It is not enough to pay sentimental tribute to the ideal family doctor, the "Marcus Welbys" of television make-believe and public yearning. We must now create the institutions and conditions to make it possible for real live doctors to be both scientists and humanists and to shift their primary attention from crisis intervention to lifetime prevention and health maintenance.

Four separate but equally important approaches are involved:

1. An increase in the quantity of doctors and other health professionals in numbers significant enough to correct the present serious imbalance in supply and demand and to relieve the growing pressures and tensions in consumer-provider relations noted in Chapters 1 and 2;

2. Rationalization of health care facilities and programs to assure optimum use of existing and future personnel;

3. Redefinition of professional roles to assure personalized care within the essential organizational matrix;

4. The strengthening and improving of financing mechanisms to make sure that no one is prevented from obtaining needed health services, preventive as well as curative, for lack of money; that there is an adequate and stable supply of funds to support a balanced health care program for all segments of the community; and that distortions in present methods of paying health personnel which tend to emphasize treatment at the expense of prevention and maintenance are corrected.

The second of these approaches will be discussed in Chapter 7, the fourth in Chapter 8. This chapter deals with points 1 and 3. Although both are equally urgent, the emphasis here is placed on point 3, assurance of personalized care, since the problem has been inadequately defined in recent discussions.

More Doctors and Other Health Professionals

From time to time, some economists and systems engineers claim that under a more rational organization of health services productivity could be increased substantially and the need for additional personnel, especially doctors, would disappear.[1] The author disagrees. Under such a reorganization, discussed in Chapter 7, the number of additional personnel needed should be less than without such reorganization, but the object of reorganization is to improve accessibility and quality as well as economy. To overemphasize the latter is to doom any reorganization effort to failure. Moreover, unless the supply of health personnel is substantially increased and more flexibility in their deployment achieved, it is doubtful that we can effect even the minimal institutional reforms necessary to bring about a meaningful rise in productivity.

It is also worth noting that, among the advanced nations, the United States has one of the lower physician/population ratios. Nine countries, Israel and eight European nations, have higher ratios than we.[2]

Finally, our dependence upon foreign medical schools for more than one-fourth of our physician licentiates each year is intolerable and must be gradually phased out. In the words of Dr. John Knowles:

> This is the only moral and practical thing to do. This means clearly that we must accelerate the expansion of existing medical schools and teaching hospitals so that we can at least double the output of physicians over the coming years.[3]

The whole broad field of education for the health professions—the changes that must be made to meet the need for both quantitative and qualitative improvements, and the many innovative programs already in progress—is beyond the scope of this work.[4] However, it is impossible to exaggerate the importance of such educational reforms if our health care needs are to be met.

Closely related to the health manpower problem, but obviously involving many other considerations, is the possibility of a civilian alternative to the military draft. A National Youth Corps, involving one or two years between high school and college for both boys and girls, would logically include a major health care component. It could help to provide much needed paraprofessional manpower and would give useful training and learning experience for hundreds of thousands of potential recruits to permanent health industry employment.

Obviously, it would also call for far-reaching adjustments and would create some problems for the health care providers. But the potential advantages—to the industry, to the nation, which is currently wasting the idealism and energy of large segments of its youth, and, most important, to the young people themselves —appear so great that it deserves immediate serious study, which might well be undertaken by Congress and the Administration. If the military draft is repealed without the establishment of some broad new civilian corps, the opportunity may be lost for a generation or more.

In any case, it will not be possible to formulate the changing educational goals without a clearer concept of the evolving health care delivery system. Too often, the alternatives are presented as simply systemization versus old-fashioned one-to-one care. In fact, neither alternative is acceptable and, as already indicated, the challenge is to harmonize the drive for rationalization with the drive for broader and more meaningful personal relations than in the past.

[1]For this and succeeding notes in this chapter, see page 96.

Three ways of dealing with the problem of personal relations will be noted: (1) revitalization of the doctor-patient relationship, (2) development of new categories of physician-surrogates, and (3) much more attention to the concept of the health care team.

Revitalization of the Doctor-Patient Relationship

The need for a personal doctor-patient relationship is widely recognized. The patient's plea for such a relationship is heard on all sides, with varying degrees of sophistication. His complaint as to inability to establish such a relationship is probably the most widely expressed criticism of medical care today, more urgent in the minds of many than even rising costs. When the two are linked together in personal experience, high cost for impersonal care, the result is often a bitterness that bodes ill for patients and providers alike. No doubt some of this criticism is the result of an oversell of the personal doctor-patient relationship, a propaganda backfire. Some of it involves nostalgia for a past that never really was, a past in which a small percentage of the population did enjoy excellent personal care, but also a past in which the vast majority was barred from such care by financial, geographic, cultural, or other barriers.

But this yearning for an ideal that was always more myth than fact is not without meaning. Partly, there is an intuitive grasping for a human being to translate into terms the patient can understand the impersonal vocabulary of the computer, the x-ray, and the blood analyzer. Partly, too, there is the instinctive realization that the patient must be viewed as a whole if effective management of his illness is to be achieved. This can only be done by a human being who can sort out and integrate all the information and advice provided by the various specialists and then translate the result into meaningful therapy for the patient. In brief, this yearning for a personal physician and a personal doctor-patient relationship, while partly nostalgic and partly the product of propaganda, has a firm basis in the realities of good medical care. It is a legitimate demand.

The problem is also recognized, at least in theory, by the medical profession—both the practitioner and the academic physician. The American Academy of General Practice and the Family Health Foundation of America have done a great deal to emphasize the need.[5] Through the Coggeshall report,[6] the Millis report,[7] and other studies, the American Medical Association and the Association of American Medical Colleges have helped publicize the need for a new specialty of family medicine. In 1969, such a specialty was officially established (Chapter 1).

It is still not clear, however, whether this new specialist will fill the gap completely. For what is involved is not only greater understanding of the socioeconomic factors involved in illness and health, and more insight into the complexities and subtleties of human relationships in an age of science, technology, and alienation, but also, and just as important, an organizational setting that makes possible the desirable relationship.

The phrase "a good doctor-patient relationship" has been so abused in recent years, as a propaganda weapon in the futile effort to stave off third-party financing, that critics believe it has lost all its meaning. If so, it is time that real content be injected into the concept. Here is a simple working definition which may be useful as a starting point: a relationship in which both the doctor and the patient feel comfortable and confident in terms of the particular demands put on them. This may seem very loose as a definition but it has to be so because medical care, like illness itself, is a complex and highly diversified affair. There is a tremendous difference in the kind of relationship expected by a teen-age boy who breaks his arm and is taken to the emergency room and that expected and needed by the terminal cancer patient.

Yet there are some common ingredients even in this vast spectrum of situations. Here are five essential characteristics, all of which happen to start with the letter "C"—competence, caring, confidence, comprehensiveness, and continuity. The first three are indispensable to any good doctor-patient relationship, regardless of how brief or simple it is.

First and most basic of all, the doctor must have competence. Second, he must have a sense of dedication to his work. He need not have any special "bedside manner" or personal charm. But he must have integrity and this applies both to his competence and his concern for the patient. If he has these two qualities, he is likely to be confident himself. The patient, in turn, is likely to sense this and have confidence in him.

For many situations, these three ingredients are enough. It is not necessary for every pathologist and every surgeon to establish a continuing or comprehensive relationship with their patients. In the effort to stress the need for comprehensiveness, it is possible to underestimate the importance of this simpler but still very important relationship.

For an increasing number of situations, however, this relatively simple relationship is no longer adequate. As the proportion of older people in the population rises, as we keep alive more and more people with serious disabilities, as the poor are given access to "mainstream" medical care and the rich have access to more health-threatening drugs and diversions, the proportion of chronic to acute illness rises, the proportion of psychosomatic illness rises, and so does the proportion of combined medical and socioeconomic problems. In all of these situations, the simple relationship based on specialized competence and integrity is no longer adequate. Such people require the two other "C's"—continuity and comprehensiveness.

At the simplest level this is evident in the case of drug incompatibilities. The patient with glaucoma has to worry about the possibly injurious effect of drugs prescribed for other conditions. The patient with both an ulcer and a kidney problem may find it hard to reconcile his medications. One man's pain reliever is another's poison. The older we get, the longer the medical history we accumulate, the more difficult it may become to balance often-conflicting therapies. Then, too, the patient's socioeconomic problems become highly relevant. It does little good to prescribe rest and "light work" to the injured longshoreman or coal miner who knows no other trade unless he can be helped to develop a new skill, or to prescribe abstinence to the alcoholic or drug addict unless he can be helped to overcome the addiction. All of these people desperately need a personal physician, one who can provide, or supervise the provision of, a regimen of care that includes both continuity and comprehensiveness.

The fact remains, however, that for a large proportion of the American people, the middle class as well as the poor, these essential ingredients of a meaningful doctor-patient relationship are conspicuously lacking. For example, a recent survey of newborn infants in two New York City health districts, one a slum, the other a middle-income area, disclosed there was no continuity of care for at least 40 percent of the babies of the white middle class, for 75 percent of the babies of the minority middle class, and for 90 percent of the babies of the minority lower class.[8]

In the effort to enable our limited number of doctors to devote more of their limited time to these aspects of patient care, every effort should be made to help them organize their work schedules more efficiently. For many, not necessarily all, this means group practice or hospital-based practice, which is more likely to provide access to the growing inventory of human and mechanical aids to diagnosis and routine therapeutic procedures, leaving the doctor more time for face-to-face discussion with the patient, for interpretation, instruction, and emotional support.

Clearly doctors should be relieved of all paper work and all mechanical chores such as injections or measurements. In the words of one physician:

> There is no doubt that nondoctors can render many of the services doctors traditionally perform in our culture. . . . An ophthalmologist prescribing glasses is over-trained for this job—by about 12 years.[9]

A 1967 survey of Regular Fellows of the American Academy of Pediatrics reported a striking contrast between the proportion of respondents now delegating patient-care tasks and those indicating they would do so if capable trained personnel were available. The vast majority said that they would hire such personnel and that this would increase the volume or improve the quality of pediatrics or both.[10]

As to the patient attitudes toward greater delegation of routine tasks to aides, *Medical Economics* recently surveyed a sample of patients with the following question: "If your doctor employed more nurses or other assistants to help him provide patient care and didn't do relatively minor things himself (routine injections and instructions, for example), how would you feel about it?"[11]

Only 18 percent of the respondents said they would dislike the arrangement; 72 percent said they wouldn't mind; and 11 percent said they would like it. Respondent attitudes were, as would be expected, closely related to their experience with competent or incompetent aides.

The medical record could be greatly improved—made more comprehensive and at the same time simpler and faster to record—on the basis of standardized, problem-oriented forms, and eventually hospital-based computerized storage and retrieval.[12]

The possibilities for more efficient use of the doctor's time, even the doctor in solo practice, are legion and are, of course, being diligently pursued by many doctors today. In too many cases, however, the net result is simply that the doctor sees more patients rather than improving the quality of the time he spends with them. This may improve his income and superficially help to satisfy some of the new demand. It does not usually improve the doctor-patient relationship and it is questionable how much the all-too-typical five- to six-minute office visit (page 9) contributes to the national health.

New Categories of Physician-Surrogates

The shortage of trained personnel is now so great and the demand so intense that all sorts of persons, trained and untrained, are being thrown into the breach. Public health nurses, social workers, and home health aides—a new category of indigenous personnel, with three to six months of training, widely used in OEO neighborhood health centers—all are helping to fill the chasm between scientific medicine and the bewildered patient.

If our society is forced to turn for a physician-surrogate to 18-year-old high school dropouts and middle-aged grandmothers who have been given three months of catch-as-catch-can training, if this is the best we can do in this affluent nation that is spending some $64 billion a year on health care, so be it. It's probably better than nothing. When a man is dying, he doesn't question the training of the hand that holds his own. It's the human warmth that counts. The ghetto mother with seven children and a persistent backache may get more practical help from an aide who can direct her to needed social services than from an orthopedic surgeon who can only report that the x-ray shows no spinal pathology.

Mini-Doctor or Maxi-Nurse?

There is really no excuse, however, for such a situation today. We have known for some years that there probably will not be enough doctors, at least as presently trained, to meet the need for personalized care. Some have suggested that the personal physician of the future should be some sort of mini-doctor with less than the standard baccalaureate plus the MD degree. There have been numerous proposals to this effect, including the suggestion for a three-year "family doctor" or "medical practitioner," and one for a "clinical associate," whose education would consist of four years of a special medical school, immediately following high school, plus one additional year of apprenticeship or internship.

Or, should we take a different route altogether? There are numerous non-MD candidates for the job. Starting with the well-known Duke University program for training ex-military corpsmen as "physicians' assistants," a number of programs of this type have recently been launched. "Medex," "surgical assistant," "orthopedic assistant," "pediatric nurse practitioner," "child health associate," "nurse physician associate," "patient care expediter," "medical service associate," "triage professional"—these are just a few of the many new titles and job categories that are struggling to be born in one place or another.[13]

In Denver, pediatric nurse practitioners, trained at the University of Colorado School of Medicine and working under the general supervision of pediatricians, are already taking care of children, both the well and the sick. In a few teaching hospitals in New York City and elsewhere, nurse-midwives are playing the same role in obstetrics. At the University of Kansas Medical Center, ambulatory care is being given in experimental "nurse clinics," with some interesting results. Patients seen in the nurse clinics report a significant reduction in the frequency of symptoms, a decrease in the number of broken appointments, and a significant increase in employment.[14] By contrast, patients seen in the regular Medical Center clinic report no change in number of symptoms and a decrease in employment. The latter group was more. critical of the care they received and more prone to shop around for other forms of health care.

The latest development in Colorado, probably the most experimental state in the nation in this respect, relates to the child health associate. She is not a nurse but a girl with five years of training after high school, including two of liberal arts, two of special pediatrics training in the medical school, and one of internship. She will be somewhere between a nurse and a doctor, with considerably more authority than the pediatric nurse practitioner. The first class started at the University of Colorado Medical School in the fall of 1969, and the state laws have been amended to permit her licensure. This could be extremely significant and might lead, for example, to a whole new category of "family health associate," helping to fill the gap between doctor and nurse with respect to general primary care.

More Attention to the Health Care Team

Thus far, there is no general agreement as to the primary purpose of the new health professions, except to help relieve the overall professional shortage. Some see them primarily as technical aides to the physician, an extension of his own specialized skills. The orthopedic assistant would clearly fall into this category. Others see them primarily as physician-surrogates, especially in the area of primary and preventive care. Obviously, appropriate educational programs and licensing requirements would differ widely depending on which of these two purposes is to be emphasized.

In fact, both are needed. But to avoid utter confusion and a serious threat to the quality of care, much more thought needs to be given to the relationship of these new job categories and training programs to each other; to the older professions—not only the doctor but, very importantly, the nurse and pharmacist whose continuing indispensable roles are often overlooked; to the very concept of the "health care team"; and to the evolving health care delivery system. To develop the new categories, one by one, and seek to license them, one by one, would, almost inevitably, do more harm than good.

The confusion, contradictions, financial strain, and general turmoil surrounding the changing role of the hospital intern and resident are well known. Less dramatic perhaps, but equally serious, is the considerable demoralization we are currently witnessing of the nursing profession, including public health nursing. For a variety of reasons, which need to be identified and publicly discussed, this important profession finds itself today in a sort of professional and organizational limbo.[15] Although salaries and working conditions have improved considerably in recent years, they are in most cases still inadequate and, as nonprofessional earnings continue to rise under the pressure of unionism, will appear increasingly out of balance. Even more important, the basic issue as to the role of the nurse in the evolving health care team remains unsettled and unsettling—to the nurse, the doctor, the hospital, and the patient. Numerous recent study commissions dealing with nursing and nursing education have still not come to grips with this problem.

The dilemma of nursing illustrates the general problem regarding the "health care team." For some years, it has been fashionable to speak of the "team," thus paying at least lip service to the essential role of the dentist, the nurse, the pharmacist, the medical social worker, the hospital administrator, and others. In a few areas teams do function effectively. Heart and brain surgeons often put together beautifully orchestrated teams of operating room personnel, from MD to scrub nurse. In some hospitals, "team nursing" has brought together the RN, the LPN, the aide, the ward clerk, and others. In the field of rehabilitation, multidisciplinary teams, designed to get the patient from the operating table back to work, have produced virtual miracles of recovery. OEO has pioneered, in some of its neighborhood health centers, with primary care teams, including doctor, public health nurse, and social worker. The military services appear to have developed some highly efficient teams utilizing the services of specially trained corpsmen, experience which, thus far, has been almost completely ignored in civilian life.[16]

Indeed, the concept of the health team remains, by and large, a figure of speech. The health professions resemble more a hierarchy than a team. Most doctors, and even nurses, are individual entrepreneurs, in work habits even if not financially. The irony is that this extreme individualism, instead of improving the patient-professional relationship, frequently makes a sound relationship impossible. The hurried, harried doctor or nurse, preoccupied with minutiae and mechanical details, cannot function as the wise, compassionate adviser. Who ever saw Marcus Welby in a hurry? What do we really mean by the health care team, especially in the area of primary care?

What is needed now is a variety of experiments along all the lines that have been suggested and others not yet thought of. These experiments should deal with the development of (1) an appropriate personal physician, with the competence, interest, and time to maintain a personal continuing and educational relationship with his patients—the sort of relationship that the fortunate minority now have with their pediatricians, internists, or obstetricians, but that is unavailable to millions; (2) an effective physician-surrogate who could handle, for those unable to achieve such a relationship with a doctor, at least part of the personal aspects of health care; and (3) appropriate health care teams to deal with various types of patient populations in various settings, institutional and noninstitutional.

While it is obviously easier to develop such teams in an institutional setting, it is not necessarily the only way. In the words of one wise doctor:

> It would be a sad commentary indeed if we find we have to have all personnel paid by the same employer to achieve the mutual respect which is really the catalyst needed to improve patient care.[17]

Regardless of setting, both the second and third categories of experiments will require simultaneous experimentation with new approaches to personnel licensing —an absolute prerequisite to solution of the growing health manpower crisis.[18]

There is reason to believe that most hospitals, doctors, nurses, and other health professionals would welcome such experiments, if responsibly planned and executed. A recent editorial in the *Archives of Internal Medicine,* entitled "Concern About Patient Care," concluded as follows:

The eventual solution to these dilemmas will not be along any one path but rather by way of the whole series of responses that entail efforts in all areas: social and psychological training, generalist emphasis, allied health personnel development. The common denominator for all these developments, however, will have to be found in a consistent concern for the degrees of satisfaction and comfort that the patient experiences. . . . A key component in the equation is the opportunity for the patient and the family to tell the physician what they think and feel as treatment progresses. In that context, the doctor-patient relationship becomes a two-way educational process. If a great many such transactions were to occur, it may well be that the lessons shared by both patients and staff would lead to the ultimate goal to which all the criticisms are being leveled, namely, to the greater concordance between the scientific excellence and the psychosocial facets of medical care.[19]

Young professionals entering the health care field today would almost certainly be delighted. Dr. George Harrell, dean of the new Pennsylvania State University College of Medicine, which specifically emphasizes family medicine, reports over 2500 applications for the 64 places available. At Duke University, Dr. Robert Howard, director of the physician's assistant program, reports nearly 100 applications a week for the 40 places available in the sixth year of that program.

Conversely, Congress and the American people should realize that it is futile to set up programs that will further increase the demand for health services unless corollary steps are taken to increase and improve the medical and other health manpower necessary to render the services.

NOTES

1. Economist Eli Ginzberg of Columbia University opposes an increase in MDs (although presumably not in other professionals) for a different reason—fear of the growing danger of over-doctoring *(Med. Econ.,* June 8, 1970, pp. 21-34). The present author shares his concern for over-doctoring, as well as his conviction that numbers alone will not cure the maldistribution. These two problems can best be dealt with by reorganization of the delivery system and by changes in methods of payment. But changes in the delivery system or methods of payment will be impossible to achieve democratically without substantial loosening of the current shortage of doctors. For a persuasive case in favor of a 50 percent rise in medical students and a 20 percent rise in dental students over the next decade, see *Higher Education and the Nation's Health,* The Carnegie Commission on Higher Education (McGraw-Hill, 1970).

2. Austria, Bulgaria, Czechoslovakia, Denmark, West Germany, Hungary, Italy and Monaco. Belgium has the same ratio, Switzerland almost the same. Sweden and Great Britain are somewhat lower. United Nations Statistical Office, Department of Economic and Social Affairs, *Statistical Yearbook* (New York, 1968), pp. 701-05.

3. Knowles, J., The physician in the decade ahead, *Hospitals, J.A.H.A.,* Jan. 1, 1970, p. 62.

4. For discussion, as of mid-1967, see, Darley, W. and Somers, A. R., Medicine, money and manpower, *New Engl. J. Med.,* Series of four articles, June 1967.

5. See, for example, *Training Family Physicians to Render Comprehensive Care.* Proceedings of a Conference of the Family Health Foundation of America, Supplement to *GP,* Aug. 1967.

6. Coggeshall, L. T., *Planning for Medical Progress Through Education* (Evanston, Ill.: Association of American Medical Colleges, 1965).

7. American Medical Association, *The Graduate Education of Physicians,* Report of Citizens Commission on Graduate Medical Education (J. S. Millis, Chairman), 1966.

8. Mindlen, R. L. and Densen, P. M., Medical care of urban infants: Continuity of care. *Amer. J. Public Health,* Aug. 1969, p. 1301.

9. Halberstam, M., *New York Times Mag.,* Nov. 9, 1969, p. 71.

10. Yankauer, A., Connelly, J. P., and Feldman, J. F., Task performance and task delegation in pediatric office practice. *Amer. J. Public Health,* July 1969, pp. 1104-16.

11. *Med. Econ.* June 8, 1970, p. 91.

12. See, for example, Weed, L. L., Medical records that guide and teach. *New Engl. J. Med.* Mar. 14, 21, 1968, pp. 593-600, 625-57. Also *Medical Records, Medical Education, and Patient Care* (Cleveland: Press of Case Western Reserve University, 1969).

13. See, for example, Kadish, J. and Long, J. W., The training of physician assistants: status and issues. *J. Amer. Med. Assn.* May 11, 1970, pp. 1047-51. Also, Light, I., Development and growth of new allied health fields. *J. Amer. Med. Assn.* Oct. 6, 1969, pp. 114-20.

14. Lewis, C. and Resnik, B., Nurse clinics and progressive ambulatory patient care. *New Engl. J. Med.* Dec. 7, 1967, pp. 1236-41. Also, Lewis, Resnik, *et al.,* Activities, events, and outcomes in ambulatory patient care. *New Engl. J. Med.* Mar. 20, 1969, pp. 645-49

15. See, for example, Bennett, L. R., Nurses may become extinct. *Nursing Outlook,* Jan. 1970, pp. 28-32.

16. See, for example, National Academy of Sciences, Ad Hoc Committee on Allied Health Personnel, *Allied Health Personnel: A Report on Their Use in the Military Services as a Model for Use in Nonmilitary Health Care Programs* (Washington, D.C., 1969). Also, Darley, W., Allied health personnel and their need for the improvement of medical care. (Editorial). *New Engl. J. Med.* Aug. 21, 1969, pp. 443-45.

17. Williams, T., Ohio Academy of General Practice, *The Patient and Allied Health Workers* (Mimeo.), p. 6. Group Health Insurance of New York, an innovative plan emphasizing family health care by solo practitioners, is hoping to initiate a demonstration project in which social services would be provided by GHI to Medicaid and other low-income patients with their records tied in to GHI's general computerized medical records—in effect, a group without walls (George Melcher, GHI President, Interview, New York City, Nov. 6, 1969).

18. For general discussion of this subject, see, Somers, A. R., *Hospital Regulation: The Dilemma of Public Policy* (Princeton University, 1969), Chap. V, Personnel licensure. Also, Riley, C. M., Univ. of Colo. School of Med., *Discussion of Licensing of Human Health Practitioners in Colorado and Proposals for Change* (Mimeo, 1968) and other publications. Also, Hershey, N., An alternative to mandatory licensure of health professionals, *Hosp. Prog.* March 1969, pp. 71-74, and other publications.

19. *Arch. Int. Med.* June 1969, p. 721.

Chapter 7

RATIONALIZATION OF COMMUNITY HEALTH SERVICES AND THE ROLE OF THE HOSPITAL

The solo medical practitioner and single community hospital facility will be as obsolete as the blacksmith within several decades. Along with them, many of the social and voluntary nonprofit agencies involved in health activities will merge, disappear, or become absorbed into larger units.

MARTIN S. ULAN
American Journal of Pharmaceutical Education (December 1968)

Until we see the delivery of medical and health care in this country as a matter of arrangements, we will make no progress. It is how you relate resources, as well as how you relate the personal components of those resources, that counts. . . . I would define the hospital of the future simply as an organization. In other words, it will no longer be seen as a beautiful structure on a hill; it will be simply a matter of arrangement. In many instances it will be the delivery of medical care by different types of individuals from different locations within a city.

RAY E. BROWN
Hospitals, J.A.H.A. (January 1, 1970)

In a country with the size and diversity of the United States, it is not surprising that no one specific method for the delivery of health services has won universal approbation. The particular form that is dominant in any given community depends on many local factors, including the socioeconomic status of the patient population; the number, quality, and organization of physicians; the presence or absence of a medical school; the organization and outreach of the community hospital; the presence or absence of neighborhood health centers, nursing homes, and other health facilities; methods of financing; and the relative role of public and private institutions.

The Ultimate Aim: Comprehensive Care for All

Despite this diversity, there is a growing consensus among providers and consumers alike that both the organization and financing of health care should be so ordered as to assure to all Americans something called "comprehensive care." It is not possible to define "comprehensive care" to the satisfaction of everyone, any more than we can define precisely what we mean by "democracy" or "freedom." It is possible to identify a number of essential conditions without which comprehensive care cannot be provided. Here are four:

99

1. Every individual must have access, as needed, without financial or other barriers, to the whole spectrum of health services—preventive, advisory, rehabilitative, and long-term care, as well as diagnostic and therapeutic—through organized referral channels that do not break the primary personal relationship, do not require unnecessary duplication of diagnostic tests or other services, and provide complete and continuous records of all medical and other health-related information.

2. Every individual must have access to a meaningful personal relationship with at least one health professional, preferably a primary physician or a specialist who can provide the necessary general coordination and continuity. Where this is not possible, he should have access to a professional physician-surrogate who would be responsible for his health records and for coordinating the various specialty services.

3. There must be enough doctors, nurses, and other health personnel to effect points 1 and 2.

4. Every physician and other health professional should be subject to an organized system of professional discipline or peer review involving the quality, quantity, and price of services rendered. Every health institution must be subject to some form of price discipline—through market competition, public regulation, or a combination of both.

Obviously, not everyone will agree with this approach to the definition of comprehensive care. Some may say it is too broad to be meaningful; others may find it too rigid. With a concept such as this it is neither possible nor necessary to achieve complete agreement. What is essential is enough consensus to enable us to move from the philosophical to the practical plane so that we can begin to determine the necessary modifications in the present delivery system or "nonsystem."

This chapter contains two proposals—(1) a redefinition of the role of the hospital as center of community health services and (2) an improved pluralistic planning and regulatory mechanism including state hospital franchisement—which could go a long way toward facilitating fulfillment of the four prerequisites and thus the achievement of community-wide comprehensive care.

The Central Role of the Hospital

Just as the hospital medical staff organization currently controls and coordinates medical practice and hospital service related to inpatients, by the end of the Seventies it will perform the same function with respect to ambulatory patients in clinics, emergency units, health centers, and in the offices of private practitioners. The efforts of hospitals and private practitioners will be more and more closely coordinated to achieve comprehensive programs of medical service.

ROBERT M. SIGMOND
Medical Economics (May 11, 1970)

An essential point must be emphasized from the outset: In referring to the hospital, we are not talking about a physical plant but about a complex social organization, including trustees, medical staff, administration, nursing service, and so forth. In Ray E. Brown's words (page 99), the hospital should now be viewed primarily as an "organizational arrangement." But what makes it different from other "organizational arrangements," for example, the Garfield system (page 110), is that it is not just an abstraction. The hospital is a living, dynamic embodiment of centuries of scientific and humanitarian efforts, an amalgam of often conflicting, but basically complementary, community and professional pressures.

It is proposed that this unique institution, which has already emerged as the principal workshop for most of the health professions and is becoming a *de facto* community health center, should now actively seek, and be officially assigned, the role of organizational catalyst, referral center, and professional monitor of the quality and quantity of care rendered not only on its own premises but throughout its community.

The proposal that it play the central role does not mean that all community health services actually would be provided within its four walls. On the contrary, the community health system of the future not only will call for fewer acute beds per capita than at present, but also will stress physical decentralization for all services except those that actually require sophisticated technical equipment and highly specialized personnel. There will be increasing emphasis on neighborhood health centers, which will be located in affluent as well as underprivileged neighborhoods, on private group practice clinics, on first-aid stations in isolated localities, on good long-term care facilities, and on home health programs.

But the hospital, as the broadest-based source of authority in terms of professional, technical, and financial resources, the site where professional needs and values and community needs and values meet and can be reconciled, will be assigned responsibility for assuring the essential functional and organizational relationships—through satellite units, affiliation agreements, inter-institutional contracts, etc.—to make the complex and interrelated system work for the entire community, on a predominantly voluntary (nongovernmental) basis.

This means that the hospital will become both the primary operational center for community health services and the primary center for comprehensive health planning at the community level. Combining of operational and planning responsibility is essential if comprehensive health planning is to be meaningful at the point of actual delivery.

Some may feel this is an unreasonable burden to place on the hospital and one for which most are not prepared in terms of experience, skills, financing, or even philosophy. It is true that many hospitals, perhaps most, are not yet prepared to meet such a challenge. But many others, including some of the large, pace-setting institutions, are clearly moving in this direction. So are the American Hospital Association,[1] the Catholic Hospital Association,[2] and many state associations. Given adequate encouragement, moral and political as well as financial, most of the industry would probably be prepared to follow suit.

Moreover, this proposal is not as revolutionary as it may first sound. Increasingly, as noted in Chapter 3, public opinion and the law are holding the hospital responsible, even legally liable, for the quality and quantity of care rendered within it. This responsibility is increasingly being assumed and, with varying degrees of effectiveness, discharged by a network of hospital-based professional review

[1]For this and succeeding notes in this chapter, see page 125.

and audit committees. Thus far, this responsibility and the system of professional review have been limited to care actually rendered on the hospital premises. It is now proposed that this responsibility be extended to care throughout the hospital's entire service area, including care rendered in satellite clinics and neighborhood health centers, mental health clinics and rehabilitation centers, nursing homes, home health programs, by visiting nurses, and even that rendered by affiliated physicians in their private offices.

The concept of grouping community health facilities around the community hospital and the latter's affiliation with a regional teaching hospital or medical center has been advocated by health care authorities for three or four decades. Such a development was implicit in the report and legislation that led to the Regional Medical Program in 1965.[3] It was explicitly recommended by the National Commission on Community Health Services in 1967.[4] Many of the nation's leading health care authorities, including Dr. Edwin L. Crosby,[5] Mark Berke,[6] Ray E. Brown,[7] Robert M. Sigmond,[8] Dr. Russel V. Lee,[9] and others[10] have urged a similar course of action.

Illustrative Projections — Circa 1976

What do the words "organizational catalyst," "referral center," and "professional monitor" mean in practice? Obviously, in a country of this size, with wide regional and cultural variations, they will mean different things in different places. At the risk of oversimplification, here are two illustrations—two imaginary hospitals operating in the context of the proposed model about five years from now. In projecting these examples, an evolutionary development has been assumed, with all this means in terms of some continuing irrationalities, rather than a drastic revolutionary overhauling of our present nonsystem—an overhauling that might well lose more than it would gain.

Mercy Community Hospital

Mercy is a typical community hospital of the mid-1970s, one of six serving a highly urbanized city of about 500,000.

Urbanton does not really need six hospitals. Three would probably be enough and more in line with the national trend to fewer, larger institutions. However, until 1971, there were seven separate hospitals in this community and the reduction to six, by merger of two, represents progress.

Mercy has about 350 beds, a first-class surgical service, an intensive care unit, a coronary care unit, and a renal dialysis unit. The department of ambulatory services includes most of the usual specialty clinics, a physical rehabilitation service, a geriatric clinic emphasizing psychiatric services, a well-developed social service, an excellent emergency department, and a first-class primary care unit. There are no inpatient pediatric or maternity services.

In addition to these central facilities, Mercy operates a 200-bed extended care facility (ECF) a few blocks away, two neighborhood health centers one mile and three miles from the hospital respectively, and an extensive home health service. It has referral agreements with two additional ECFs, several nursing homes, and a community mental health center.

Most of its nonprofessional services—laundry, dietary, housekeeping, business operations—and most of the routine laboratory work are provided through a multi-hospital corporation contracting with the six hospitals.

The medical staff consists of approximately 150 physicians, about 50 of whom are full-time. These include the medical director, director of professional education, director of community medicine, and chiefs of all the major services; radiology, pathology, anesthesiology, physical medicine, and psychiatry departments *in toto;* and the staffs of the emergency department, primary care unit, and the two satellite neighborhood health centers.

Most of the doctors have their offices in the medical arts building next door to the hospital and owned by it. The largest suite is occupied by the Mercy Medical Group—a separate organization of 35 physicians. The rest of the building is occupied by doctors in varying degrees of combination, mostly two- or three-man partnerships. Nearly all—except for the obstetricians and pediatricians—have their primary affiliation with Mercy, although many have joint appointments in other hospitals as well.

Mercy's primary concern is patient care, but it has also become an important clinical teaching center. It is affiliated with Metropolitan University Hospital, about 50 miles away. Thanks to this affiliation, Mercy has an organized referral system for the superspecialties, easy consultation with the staff of University Hospital, close working relations with respect to its residency programs, and even an undergraduate program for fourth-year medical students interested in community medicine. This affiliation, plus the hospital's vastly increased interest in community medicine, have enabled it to obtain a majority of U.S.-trained house staff for the past few years, a situation that never prevailed in the 1960s.

Mercy's diploma school of nursing was discontinued several years ago, but it cooperates closely with a nearby community college in providing the clinical experience for a new three-year nursing school and it also conducts numerous additional courses for LPNs, nursing aides, and various specialized technicians. The director of professional education, who presides over these extensive educational activities, is one of the busiest men on the staff.

Mercy's patient population is still not defined as precisely as some planners would like to see. Nevertheless, a pretty clear *de facto* service or target area has gradually emerged, particularly as a result of clearer identification of the community's primary care doctors with a single institution. Since not all the hospitals provide all services, however, there is necessarily some crossing of geographical boundaries.

The policy of institutional specialization was hotly debated for several years. There were community leaders as well as doctors who felt that every hospital should have a maternity and pediatric service, a cobalt unit, a dialysis unit, an emergency department, in effect the whole gamut of hospital services. Eventually those who favored partial specialization prevailed. Mercy reluctantly gave up its inpatient pediatric and maternity services in return for recognized preeminence in geriatrics and the only dialysis unit in Urbanton. It continues to provide ambulatory pediatric and maternity care through its department of community health, but patients with serious illnesses requiring hospital admission are referred to the Good Neighbor

Hospital, only a few miles away, whose facilities and staff have specialized in these services. As *quid pro quo,* Mercy's dialysis unit and geriatric clinic serve the entire community.

Today, several years after the somewhat traumatic realignment of programs, both physicians and community appear generally pleased with the results. Better services are being provided at less cost than would otherwise have been the case. In the late 1960s, Mercy's OB service was running an occupancy of about one-third, Good Neighbor's about one-half. Today, the latter's OB rate averages close to 80 percent—about as high as a maternity service can be expected to operate effectively.

Costs at Mercy are not low. Hospital costs have continued to rise (Chapter 3). Fortunately, however, methods of financing care have also continued to develop, so that this high price is virtually never borne by an individual patient at the time of illness. After several years of heated debate and mounting pressure from both providers and consumers, Congress has adopted a form of national health insurance, providing compulsory coverage for virtually the entire population. However, consumers are permitted a considerable range of choice as to the type of coverage they prefer, and a number of voluntary carriers work with the providers in designing and operating such programs and competing for public favor.

The more affluent of Mercy's patients continue to rely on traditional types of insurance, especially the combination of basic hospital coverage and major medical. Under these plans, physicians are still paid on a fee-for-service basis. The majority of patients, however, are now covered by a new type of prepayment plan, modeled somewhat after the Kaiser Foundation Health Plan and also being sold by a number of other carriers and Health Maintenance Organizations (Chapter 4). Under its HMO contracts, Mercy Hospital agrees to provide subscribers with all necessary hospital and medical services for a flat monthly fee. So far as medical services are involved, some, for example those in neighborhood health centers, are provided by salaried doctors. For others, the hospital subcontracts with the Mercy Medical Group. Inpatient maternity and pediatric services and highly specialized services such as open heart or brain surgery are purchased by Mercy on behalf of these patients from other institutions with which it has referral agreements.

The financial arrangements are complicated and probably more expensive than if provided under a single national Medicare plan. However, they are clearly in line with the traditional preference of the providers of care in the United States for pluralistic financing, no matter how complicated, rather than outright government operation. In any case, the institution of a capitation or a flat fee-per-person payment for hospital and medical costs and their integration into a single program have helped considerably to make doctors more cost conscious, to force hospitals to greater managerial efficiency, and generally to restrain the rise in costs to bearable dimensions.

Metropolitan University Hospital

Metropolitan University Hospital is one of the nation's hundred best and largest teaching hospitals, the primary teaching arm of a first-rate medical school. With 800 beds it has virtually every major specialty and superspecialty. It also has a large and active department of community and family medicine, which is largely responsible for administering the network of affiliations with community hospitals and other community health facilities and programs.

Like Mercy, it also has an active ambulatory service and several neighborhood health centers. Unlike at Mercy, however, these are operated primarily as research, teaching, and demonstration units. They are relatively small and deliberately focused on the most difficult patient populations within reasonable access. For example, one center is located in a skid row area, where drug addiction and alcoholism, combined with multiple socioeconomic problems, present University's department of community medicine and department of drug and alcohol studies with abundant "teaching material" while providing the inhabitants of this area with as good care as can be found anywhere in the country. Patient care for this grossly atypical population is heavily subsidized by a new Institute of Community Medicine in the National Institutes of Health.

The ambulatory center in University Hospital itself seeks to present students and faculty with a typical cross section of the population. The number it serves, however, is deliberately restricted to a number that can be dealt with at the inevitably slower pace required for patient care in an academic setting. This also helps to minimize any town-gown conflict. The costs are paid in the same way as at Mercy—partly by traditional insurance, partly by capitation plans, but in all cases with an educational subsidy. Thus the carriers and subscribers are not charged the extra cost of academic care. The patient population is largely self-selected and comes from a relatively large area of the metropolis.

University's residents and interns, as well as graduate students in public health and hospital administration and even a substantial number of undergraduates, are rotated among several of the affiliated community hospitals, like Mercy. This is particularly true of those who are specializing in community or family medicine. Conversely, residents from the community hospitals come into University at frequent intervals for conferences, grand rounds, and for a two-week residency each year. The interchange between house staff and faculty in the two types of institutions has been enriching to both and has improved the quality of patient care available in the entire area.

Primary Care Facilities

To complete the picture, one would have to give similar vignettes illustrating the organization and work of institutions that are smaller and less sophisticated professionally than Mercy Hospital. Depending on the cultural and physical geography of the area and region, these might include a small rural hospital, a neighborhood health center in a large urban area, a private group practice clinic, an emergency first-aid station in a sparsely populated region or in a seasonal resort area, whose primary facility might be a helicopter or a Piper Cub, a college infirmary, a small industrial hospital in the mining or lumbering fields, or any number of other types of primary care units where emergency services must be provided on a standby basis but where the chief requirement in any serious situation is quick transfer to a fully equipped hospital.

The diversity of such institutions precludes doing justice to this echelon of the developing health care system. More will be said about the neighborhood health center below. It should be clear, however, that such primary care institutions are vitally important links in the total delivery picture if all Americans are to be provided with comprehensive health care. The time for wishful thinking that we can persuade good young doctors to move into such areas on a solo basis is already long past. By the mid-1970s, all efforts should be concentrated on linking these primary outposts of care to our urban hospital system. Simultaneously, the urban hospitals must rise to the challenge of assuming responsibility for these units by developing mutually beneficial satellite arrangements.

The Community Hospital as an Educational Institution

One aspect of the proposed model deserves special consideration—the use of the community hospital as an educational resource in achieving the quantity and quality of personnel needed to assure the kind of personalized care discussed in Chapter 6. The following discussion comes from Dr. Ward Darley, former Executive Director, Association of American Medical Colleges:[11]

> I cannot conceive of an organization of community health services that could get along without the hospital at its core. The hospital medical staff is the community's principal guarantor of good patient care. If these staffs function as they should (perhaps it would be better to say as they could), there is no reason why the peer judgments of the quality of patient care could not be extended from the hospital itself into the community, doctors' offices, etc.
>
> Even if such extension is not in the direct line of staff authority it could come about indirectly, provided the staff took part in the proper kinds of continuing education. By "continuing education" I mean educational programs based upon the peer identification of gaps in the quality of patient care and then the development of educational programs directly aimed at correcting these gaps. Depending upon the circumstances, these programs would be aimed at the whole staff, part of the staff, or even a single individual. The continuation of staff membership should depend upon participation in this educational activity and also upon demonstration that said education has corrected the difficulty. The Association of Hospital Directors of Medical Education is rapidly paving the way to produce the kind of people that can head the kind of educational programs of which I speak.
>
> Of basic relevance is the development of hospital records that can be used for teaching and learning as well as the evaluation of patient care. Dr. Lawrence L. Weed of the University of Vermont is well along with this development, and he and people he has trained are now available to help any hospital staff learn how to do this.[12]
>
> The standard format of these records could be used by all hospitals in a given community and by physicians in their offices. The result would be records that would mean the same thing to different people and pave the way for allied health personnel to fill identified areas of responsibility, as members of a patient-care team headed by physicians, and making proper entries on the chart so that the doctor or anyone else can quickly ascertain the patient's situation at any given point in time.

The implications of this type of continuing education and record keeping go far beyond the medical staff. If the staff can really learn something about teaching and learning, it is then in a position to play an effective role in the education of nurses (all kinds, at all levels) and other health personnel. In the expansion of such educational efforts, teaming up with junior colleges (even high schools) and liberal arts colleges would be a natural. Also, the hospital could expect to qualify for internships and residencies and even clerkships for medical students. The student could be assigned to a qualified member of the staff as preceptor and given a great experience in the continuing care of patients, following the patient from office to hospital to home, thus developing an understanding of the natural history of disease —and of health.

The involvement of students (medical, nursing, and others) in home care would be greatly facilitated—particularly if patients who need such care could be discharged from the hospital to their homes but kept on the hospital census. The hospital could then send whatever equipment might be necessary to the patient's home, instruct the family how to care for the patient, and have its personnel (interns, residents, nurses) follow the patient in his home. Then if rehospitalization is needed, a second admission and the setting up of a new record would not be necessary.

I would also make a plea that extended care facilities and nursing homes be placed under the administrative and professional arm of the hospital—upon a nonprofit basis—and that hospital-based personnel render care much on the same basis as I have suggested for home care.

Coming back to the hospital as an educational institution, I see great possibilities in the area of public education. It could be the "schoolhouse" for part of a national program of consumer health education, an important local terminal in any national network that might be established. But a good part of the program should be "homemade" so that the "student group" will feel that it has personal and community relevance.

Given the proper space, equipment, and personnel—physicians, nurses, social workers, dietitians, etc.—the hospital could provide public lectures or courses on how to use the community's health and medical care facilities, accident prevention, dietary management, etc. This kind of activity would easily provide a bridge to patient care by having physicians assign selected patients to classes in weight control, management of diabetes, ulcer, etc. The activity could go further in that doctors could assign selected patients to group therapy for emotional problems, drug addiction, alcoholism, etc.

The community hospital could well serve as the usual point of entry into a community's system of medical care. . . . The principal innovation here would be the multiphasic screening clinic. The staff physician could tell new patients (except in real emergencies) to come to him after they have gone through this clinic. After the doctor receives the screening report, he would contact the patient for a thorough review of the findings, also a history and physical examination of his own. Multiphasic screening operated by the hospital would carry great implications for extending health and medical care into the area of discovery, evaluation, and management of asymptomatic disease; also into programs of health protection as well as health education.

The hospital could also play a key role as a place where the data necessary to the evaluation of patient care can be concentrated, analyzed, interpreted, and used to develop periodic environmental inventories and morbidity profiles. The input would come from patient records, multiphasic screening records, the doctors' offices, community health and welfare agencies, etc.

I do not know what the future of the county health department will be. If the community hospital functions as it could, it might house such departments or the kind of activity they now perform. I doubt if the health department survives for long as we now know it. Mortality figures, the darlings of such departments, can no longer serve as the major index of national or community health. It is the community's morbidity profile that is important, and as these profiles are compared from year to year much will be learned about the condition of the community's health.

There are, naturally, debatable details in Dr. Darley's proposal. Perhaps the most exciting thing about it is that it effectively meshes the two important concepts of systemization and personalization. Such a rationalization of regional and community patient care and educational facilities and programs not only assures better patient care but the opportunity to educate the next generation of health personnel in the personal aspects of patient care. Thus the "system," far from destroying personal care, provides the essential "organizational infrastructure" upon which such care can be based.

The practical implementation of such a model is already under way in Illinois, where Dr. George Miller of the University of Illinois College of Medicine is developing programs in medical education, at both the graduate and undergraduate levels, utilizing eight community hospitals in Peoria and Rockford.[13]

Allocating the Costs More Equitably

There is another important advantage to the proposed model—a more equitable social accounting and more rational allocation of costs. With respect to hospital costs there are two basic facts that must be kept in mind if we are to come to grips with this seemingly intractable problem:

1. The more cooperative and successful a hospital is in limiting admission to serious cases, in holding length of stay down to the absolute minimum, and otherwise fulfilling the demands of the planners, the higher its per diem costs will inevitably go.

2. From the point of view of social accounting the only way this situation can be dealt with intelligently is to average the costs of this increasingly expensive, specialized institution with the less expensive satellite and affiliated institutions. If this were done, the inevitably high costs of the inpatient unit could be absorbed in total community costs just as the inevitably high costs of the hospital's intensive care unit are averaged in the costs of the institution as a whole. This is only possible, however, in a system that is rationalized—not only organizationally but financially.

Another obvious advantage would be the reduced unit costs of many laboratory and other services made possible by the greater volume. For example, the current cost of analyzing blood samples varies from dollars to pennies, depending in large part on volume. Moreover, high-volume use makes possible not only more economical operation but more sophisticated equipment. Machines are already in existence which can quickly and inexpensively (given a reasonably high volume) draw a comparative chemical profile of an apparently normal person from a fluid sample, enabling the doctor to identify or even head off a lifetime of ailments in advance. At the present time, however, many hospitals and clinics say they do not have the volume to keep even the standard automatic blood analyzer efficiently in use.

The key to progress in this respect appears to lie in the increasing integration or coordination of separate hospital, medical, and other health care costs into a single total community-wide accounting system. The Kaiser model—comprehensive prepaid group practice (Chapter 4 and below)—is one approach. The proposed new Health Maintenance Organization is another. We come back to the question of financing in Chapter 8.

Alternative Paths to Comprehensive Care

Obviously, the franchised hospital is not the only possible model for achieving comprehensive care.* Others have been proposed, with impressive sponsorship, and should be carefully studied. On close analysis, however, it appears that there are not many serious alternatives.

Two theoretical possibilities may be dismissed forthwith. At one time, it appeared that the central role in community health care—at least the planning and coordinating role if not the actual provision of services—could be assumed by the local health department. This is no longer even a theoretical possibility. Large portions of the country simply lack a municipal or county health department. Where such departments do exist, they have, with a few notable exceptions,[14] limited themselves to public health matters, ignoring the much larger area of nongovernmental services.

In New York City and several other large urban centers municipal hospitals still provide most of the health care available to large segments of the poor. Inadequately financed, inadequately staffed, almost totally lacking in amenities, these hospitals have been increasingly criticized by professionals and consumers alike. Many are now in a real state of crisis.[15] Efforts are being made to upgrade them, through such devices as the new Health and Hospitals Corporation of New York. Significantly, however, such efforts usually draw the institutions away from city hall and toward the voluntary sector. In the end, it is the hospital, *as a hospital,* that is a rallying point for both professionals and consumers, not the hospital as an outpost of the city health department.

A few ardent supporters of organized medicine appear to believe that the county medical societies could play this role. This is equally unrealistic. Most of the societies have shown as little interest or competence in community health affairs

---

*The AHA's "Ameriplan," with its concept of the Health Care Corporation (HCC), was published in November 1970, too late for analysis in this study. Although the terminology is different, the HCC shares many characteristics with the concept of the franchised hospital. See the Report of a Special Committee on the Provision of Health Services, *Ameriplan—A Proposal for the Delivery and Financing of Health Services in the United States* (Chicago: The Association, 1970).

as the health departments have shown in the problems of the voluntary sector. Both types of organization have disqualified themselves by the narrowness of their interests and their failure to realize that the delivery system of the future must be an amalgam of public and private enterprise, of provider and consumer interests.

The Garfield "System"

Another model, which has attracted a good deal of attention lately, turns out to be not alternative but complementary. This is Dr. Sidney R. Garfield's carefully charted patient care "system" set forth in the April 1970 issue of *Scientific American*. Drawing on the Kaiser experience, of which he was one of the founding fathers, but going far beyond it, Dr. Garfield proposes an ambitious model with heavy emphasis on prevention and the use of paramedical personnel.

His first concern is to find an effective regulator of patient entry into the health care system to substitute for the physician's fee, which he considers a serious barrier to early entry and preventive care. The proposed new regulator would be a computerized health-testing service. After health testing, the patient would be referred, as appropriate, to one of three types of program and facility—health care (health education and prevention, counseling, and so forth), sick care (diagnosis and treatment of the acutely ill), or preventive maintenance (care of the chronically ill who require routine treatment, monitoring, and follow-up).

Three of the four modalities—health testing, health care, and preventive maintenance—could, according to Dr. Garfield, be provided entirely by paramedical staff under medical supervision. Only one modality—sick care—would require primarily medical staff and it, too, would be assisted by paramedical personnel. Dr. Garfield claims the system would be much more economical to operate, not only in terms of dollars but also of even scarcer medical manpower.

As thus described and depicted in the charts, the Garfield model is an abstraction —a "system" of interrelated care modalities apart from any specific institutional setting and totally lacking any human or managerial motivating force, financial, political, or other. In his text, however, Dr. Garfield is more concrete:

> In the system being proposed a central medical center, well staffed and equipped, would provide sick care. It could have four or five "outreach" neighborhood clinics, each providing the three primarily paramedical services: health testing, health care, and preventive maintenance.

In practice, therefore, it turns out that the "central medical center" or "hospital" would be the institutional and organizational focus of his system with the testing, preventive, and maintenance activities provided in satellite clinics. Thus there is no inherent conflict between this proposal and the hospital-based model presented in this chapter.

There is, however, in the opinion of this author, overemphasis in the Garfield proposal on structural formality and some unnecessary rigidities. Real-life patients will never be willing or able to "flow" as neatly as Dr. Garfield would like. Neither will real-life doctors be willing to work exclusively within the confines of his neatly drawn compartments. The personal element in health care is simply ignored. Nevertheless, his systems approach, with its emphasis on "patient flow," has contributed an important new dimension to our evolving delivery system. In a modified and humanized form, it could be assimilated into the hospital-based model and help to strengthen the preventive and maintenance aspects.

The Cronkhite-OEO Model

In April 1970, Governor Francis W. Sargent of Massachusetts announced, with considerable publicity, the launching of a new health care program for Boston's poor, under the direction of Dr. Leonard Cronkhite, Director, Children's Hospital Medical Center of Boston, and supported by a number of leading Boston businessmen and hospitals.[16] The Governor described the plan as follows:

> The target population size for our proposed system would be approximately 300,000 people. They would be served by their own comprehensive program which would include neighborhood health centers, hospitals, nursing homes, and a home care plan, all under a single management. The cornerstone of this system is the primary, or family care center, established where people need them—in neighborhoods and communities. . . . We are designing the typical neighborhood center to serve 15 to 25 thousand people.

> These centers will accept total responsibility for providing comprehensive, personal, health services for the men, women, and children within their service areas, on a 24-hour-a-day basis. They will have the ability to select the method of care needed by the sick patient, not whatever type of care happens to be covered by an insurance policy, as now exists. The care will be offered in such a way that one physician or medical team takes full responsibility for the total care of the patient and his family. The centers will focus on health education and *preventive* medical care, in order to keep people from becoming ill in the first place. They will provide first aid and dispensary services, thus answering many of the needs for those citizens who have been obliged to seek care in our already overcrowded and much higher-priced hospital emergency rooms. They will also provide a wide range of diagnostic and therapeutic services, including dental care, and—when necessary—will refer patients requiring more complex treatment to the appropriate hospital facilities.

Governor Sargent then stated that he was appointing a special committee, headed by Dr. Cronkhite, "to define precisely the management vehicle needed to accomplish this program. This vehicle should not be government itself but something akin to a nonprofit corporation."

In point of fact, despite all the publicity, the Cronkhite plan is a modest one, limited to some 300,000 of Boston's poor. Dr. Cronkhite himself has made no claim to a national model, although some admirers have. What it appears to represent is a refined formulation of the basic OEO neighborhood health center concept. With 49 such centers now funded, and 29 additional centers funded by HEW with Section 314(e) money but along lines similar to the OEO centers, it is clear that the OEO-Cronkhite model, whatever the appropriate name, has already become a significant factor in the evolving health care delivery system. Its most important features may be identified as follows:

> 1. It is directed at a disadvantaged population living in a strictly defined geographic area.

2. The programmatic focus is on primary care and the organizational or institutional focus on a primary care unit—neighborhood health center, family health center, etc.

3. Funding, at least in the early years, is almost entirely through government. Although some plans, such as Dr. Cronkhite's, hope for eventual prepayment, all have started on the basis of free care to recipients, with revenue derived primarily from government grants, secondarily from Medicaid and Medicare.

4. Heavy emphasis is placed on the development and use of nonprofessional, indigenous personnel, and on involvement of "the community" in program planning and operation.

5. The hospital is not generally viewed as part of the system. While its essentiality for acute care is acknowledged, it is generally assumed that this can be provided in emergencies on a "backup basis," without the necessity for close organizational or financial ties.

6. Physicians, in most instances, are salaried. Institutions are paid—or subsidized—on the basis of costs.

7. No one is forced to come to a center. For the target population, however, "free choice" is not, at the moment, of paramount importance. Within the center, patients or sometimes whole families are usually assigned to a health care team—doctor, nurse, social worker, home health aide, etc.

The advantages of this model may be readily identified. For millions of poor Americans, who have traditionally had to rely on indigent clinics or the nearest GP willing to take them on a more or less charity basis, the Cronkhite-OEO health center obviously represents a big step forward—in access, quality, and, equally important, in a sense of involvement or participation in health care decisions affecting their lives and welfare.

There is another advantage. Since middle-class consumers and "mainstream" providers are generally not involved, or only peripherally so, they feel less threatened by this development than by one that touches the entire community. Thus, it may prove easier to establish a totally new neighborhood health center than it would be to improve the ambulatory services in the community hospital or to alter the board of governors of the hospital. In a time of intense racial and urban crisis, these are not inconsiderable advantages.

In evaluating the general direction for the future, however, the drawbacks to this approach must also be clearly faced. While the advantages are mostly short-term, the disadvantages are mostly long-term. First, assuming that the goal is true comprehensive care, calling for fulfillment of the four prerequisites set forth at the beginning of this chapter, it is highly doubtful that the OEO-Cronkhite model meets this test.

First, there is a clear break in continuity between the primary health center services and those required when the patient must be hospitalized, even in maternity cases. In many instances, this break would be as complete as that which usually occurs when a patient from an indigent clinic is admitted as an inpatient, and is also suggestive of the traditional British dichotomy between general practice and hospital care, an historical anachronism which the British themselves are now trying to correct.[17] As European experience indicates, the effort to play down or ignore the hospital simply will not work. It remains the *de facto* center of community health care and simply must be dealt with as such. To attempt to build two competing systems—one for primary care, the other for hospital care—will inevitably result in higher costs and lower quality for both.

The fourth prerequisite also appears inadequately met. Peer review of a sort is provided in many of the neighborhood health centers by their own staff. In the beginning, idealism and the appeal of novelty and competitive salaries are likely to attract a number of excellent young doctors and other health professionals. But in time, separation from the mainstream, especially the hospital's review mechanisms, and financing difficulties will almost surely lead to second-rate care. This was the history of the union health center movement in the 1940s and 1950s.

Finally, the long-run financing of the community health centers presents a serious problem. They are almost completely outside the reach of private health insurance, and little or no effort is being made to bring them into that reach (Governor Sargent's statement represents a welcome exception in this respect). If and as the centers are extended across the country to all the indigent and medically indigent, by means of direct grants, Medicaid payments, and so forth, as many as 40 to 50 million Americans, nearly one-fourth of the population, could eventually be receiving "free" care in this manner.

At that point, it could be assumed that the other three-fourths would become resentful of having to pay for their own care, directly or through insurance or taxes, while supporting free care for the other one-fourth through taxes. Either the free care would have to be discontinued, or it would have to be made available to the entire population. In other words, we would then be committed to an eventual national health service supported by general taxes rather than a national health insurance scheme based primarily on contributory financing.

It is not easy to reconcile these short-run gains and long-run dangers in the OEO-Cronkhite proposals. As short-run therapy for a major crisis, they have clearly played a valuable role. To continue with large doses of the same therapy could be counterproductive. The answer appears to lie in reconciliation of the many positive aspects of this model with the hospital-based model. As one element in a community-wide health care system, an element uniquely appropriate for disadvantaged populations but increasingly applicable to the affluent as well, the neighborhood health center could and should emerge as one of the major institutions in United States medical care. But standing alone, leaving the citadel of care and costs and the great majority of the population untouched, it could end up doing more harm than good.

The Kaiser Model

The second real alternative is Kaiser. The major elements of this successful private program, with its two million members, were described in Chapter 4. Widely acclaimed by health care planners, economists, and informed journalists,[18] it represents, in this author's opinion, the most original and important contribution to the delivery of health services made by this nation during the past 25 years.

Comparing its major features with those of the OEO-Cronkhite model, the following contrasts emerge:

1. It is directed at a cross section of the population living in a geographic area, but without the rigid geographic or income limits required for OEO centers.

2. Something approaching the whole spectrum of comprehensive care is provided (although specific elements such as dental care or extended mental health benefits are not available) under coordinated management and funding. There is no special emphasis on primary care but neither is it discouraged as under the fee-for-service system.

3. Funding is almost entirely private, with respect both to capital and operating costs. Unlike most other nonprofit hospitals in the United States, Kaiser hospitals have been financed out of operating surplus.

4. Paramedical personnel are used more than in conventional practice, but probably less than in the OEO centers. There is very little community involvement. Only in the past year or two have a few public or community representatives been elected to the governing board.

5. The hospital is clearly viewed as the center of the delivery system. Physicians' offices and clinics are either in a hospital or a satellite clinic. However, the real heart of the Kaiser system is the insurance plan. Both hospitals and medical groups depend on the plan for their income and for capital expansion.

6. Physicians are organized in a separate legal entity, a group, and contract with the plan to provide services for a fixed fee per enrollee per year, regardless of the amount of services provided. The amount available for payment to physicians is related to the amount required to pay hospitals. Hence, the much publicized incentive to hold down use, especially hospital use.

7. All enrollees are given a periodic choice of joining, or remaining in, the Kaiser plan or some more conventional alternative, such as Blue Cross-Blue Shield. Within the plan, members may choose their own personal doctor, who refers them to specialists as needed.

With its broad, community-wide orientation, a substantial degree of consumer free choice, effective integration of most major hospital and ambulatory services, effective managerial controls combined with considerable provider freedom, and the well-documented lesser use of expensive hospital care and lesser costs, there are many today who believe the Kaiser model is the ideal for the United States as a whole.

There are, however, a number of considerations that give pause to this conclusion. First, there is the basic fact that less than four percent of the population now belongs to a Kaiser-type plan (Table 2). Kaiser itself, the giant of the group, has less than one percent. While it is true that state laws, medical society regulations and prejudices, and hospital discrimination were, historically, very important in inhibiting the growth of prepaid group practice, it is also a fact that the gradual, although still incomplete, erosion of these restrictions and considerable positive encouragement from the federal government and informed public opinion have not been accompanied by any dramatic expansion.

Major causes for the continuing poor showing in this regard probably include the sellers' market for physicians' services—resulting in high earnings no matter how inefficient the practice and discouraging organizational innovation, a major reason for the emphasis placed by this author on the need for expanding physician manpower; the lack of enough managerial talent and start-up money for those interested in emulating the Kaiser example; the existence of some plans of this type which have not been so efficient or successful as Kaiser; and the fear of many consumers of becoming locked into a health care system about whose quality they are doubtful.

In any case, it is clear that not all patients or all doctors would be happy in this type of setting. This means that there is no democratic way that the Kaiser model could be imposed on the entire country. To impose it in any other way would be unthinkable and would clearly defeat its purpose. One of the prime secrets of Kaiser's success has been its insistence on a large degree of free choice on the part of its members, through the provision for periodic renewal or withdrawal from membership. If no alternative were available, however, and if the entire population were simply divided up among a series of Kaiser-type plans, such choice would not be available and consumers would be effectively locked in.

In the projection of Mercy Community Hospital, earlier in this chapter, it was suggested that prepaid group practice might well become the majority pattern for the future. But it was also stressed that minority patterns could, and even should, be encouraged to coexist with prepaid group practice, thus providing the discipline of competition on all types. Such competitive coexistence could be reconciled with cost and quality controls, however, only if some universally acceptable institution assumes responsibility for general coordination. This institution, it was suggested, should be the franchised hospital.

After examining all other possibilities, it appears that the omnipresent hospital, despite present shortcomings, remains the only generally available community institution with the potential capacity of assuring the provision of comprehensive care to all Americans. Both the Kaiser and OEO-Cronkhite models have made great contributions to the evolving delivery system but neither has the potential for universality, at least for the foreseeable future. On the other hand, with these two innovative concepts assimilated into a community-wide system, further enriched by Dr. Garfield's emphasis on prevention and health maintenance, coordinated by an appropriately reorganized hospital, adequately financed, and tied into an effective planning and regulatory mechanism, the possibility of developing a delivery system that could bring order out of the present chaos and assure something approaching comprehensive care to all Americans is bright indeed. Such a development would also help to facilitate a true social accounting of health care costs, thus making possible more rational allocation of those costs. It would also help to preserve, to the maximum feasible degree, voluntary control over health care services.

Moving from Here to There

Assuming the desirability of this approach to the rationalization of community health services, how can it be achieved? How to persuade the now-independent nursing homes, neighborhood centers, rehabilitation centers, and other institutions to accept the leadership of the hospital in their community? How to persuade the doctors to organize themselves primarily around the hospital? How to persuade the hospital itself to take on this burdensome and largely thankless task? And, where it is willing to do so, how to make sure that it is competent to do so? First of all, how to define "community" for the purpose of health care organization? (Questions of financing are postponed to Chapter 8.)

There are no simple or single answers to any of these questions. The only simple fact is a negative one: If the voluntary institutions do not agree among themselves on some method of achieving rationalization, it will be imposed from outside, simply because of costs. This will, almost certainly, be the beginning of the end of the voluntary system.

In any case, it cannot be done on a completely voluntary basis. Autonomy is never yielded easily. Some degree of compulsion is inevitable.[19] The degree of compulsion, the way in which it is applied, the effect on the voluntary institutions, and the net result in terms of effective community health services will all differ markedly depending on the nature of the regulatory process. Thus, the choice is not between complete voluntarism and government intervention. The choice is between a pluralistic regulatory system, designed to retain as much local initiative and private enterprise as possible but bringing in government at certain essential points—what Walter McNerney aptly calls "selective intervention"—and a regulatory system imposed almost totally by the federal government.

A Pluralistic Planning and Regulatory System
for Community Health Services

> Is not the greatest safeguard for the voluntary system a planning process with teeth in it?
>
> MARK BERKE
> *Presidential inaugural address,*
> *American Hospital Association* (1970)

What are the key elements in a workable pluralistic system? To this author there appear to be seven:

1. **The state hospital franchise.** The principal instrument for assuring the availability of comprehensive care—as defined at the beginning of this chapter— to the entire population, community by community throughout the nation, would be the state hospital franchise. The object of the franchise is to make certain that there is, in every community, an organization with the responsibility and capability for planning, delivering or coordinating, and monitoring the range of programs and services which make up the comprehensive care spectrum.

A hospital could choose to operate without a franchise. Without it, however, the hospital would not be eligible for federal, state, or local tax exemptions, for publicly funded grants or loans, or for participation in Medicare, Medicaid, and other publicly funded patient care programs. With such a franchise, it would be eligible for these advantages and would be responsible for coordinating all the health care provided by licensed physicians and other practitioners and by all licensed health facilities in its community. The franchise would be renewable periodically, say every two years.

There are, admittedly, drawbacks in use of the word "franchise." Although used in the health care field for a decade or more—the term was first popularized by Ray E. Brown, one of the nation's leading hospital authorities, around 1960, and he is still its advocate—there is no generally accepted definition. Even in its commercial usage, the term has been discredited in the past few years due to the irresponsibility of some franchise operators.

Use of the older concept of "hospital licensing" is not ruled out if it could be expanded to include the positive requirements for the franchise, indicated above, and adequately tied in with regional and federal activities. A few states—Michigan, for example—appear to be moving in this direction with an expanded concept of licensing. Equally important, many states, under the leadership of the AHA, are moving toward the requirement of a state "certificate of need" before any hospital or nursing home can expand substantially. Rather than struggle with the probable continuation of vastly different concepts of licensing in the different states, however, it would appear easier and simpler to arrive at a workable definition of "franchising," or even invent a new term, perhaps "chartering."

The minimal requirements for an acceptable hospital franchise could be defined in federal law, for federal tax exemption, participation in federal programs, and other purposes (see below), with each state left free to add such additional requirements as it sees fit. The term "license" could then be reserved for professional and institutional providers of health care, other than hospitals, and for hospitals that choose to operate without the privileges and responsibilities inherent in the franchise.

Whatever the term finally used, the concept of the franchise, suitably modified to fit the health care field, appears to offer a viable compromise between complete voluntarism and government operation. It is more relevant to a nonprofit institution such as a hospital than the concept of a public utility. The latter aims primarily to correct profiteering, which is not relevant to the voluntary hospital. The franchise, on the other hand, aims primarily to oblige the hospital to take on certain defined responsibilities for a defined area in return for defined financial advantages, and to withhold public support and privileges from institutions that are unwilling or unable to assume the responsibilities the community deems essential.

In other words, the franchise offers a device for harmonizing our traditions of local autonomy and private initiative with the degree of public control necessary to assure meeting public needs.

Would the for-profit hospitals be able to continue under the franchise system? In theory, yes. The system is not concerned with corporate structure *per se*. It is concerned with the optimum use of scarce resources. If a for-profit institution were willing to assume the burdens of a community franchise and could satisfy the regional and state authorities that it could do the job, there should be no reason why it should not obtain a franchise. On the other hand, if such an institution wishes to operate outside the franchise system altogether, without Medicare, Medicaid, or any other government money, it should also be permitted to do so. However, if manpower shortages became too acute, the nonfranchised hospital's license would have to be reconsidered.

2. **A workable way of defining "community."** Health planners have talked rather glibly, for some years, of "community health services" and of providing health care to "a defined patient population." But there has been virtually no discussion of how to define a "community" or a "patient population." In single-hospital communities there should be no special problem unless the one hospital had traditionally shown itself to be particularly unresponsive to community needs. In most cases, such a situation could be corrected under conditions of the franchise. In some rural areas, where there is no acceptable hospital to take on the responsibilities of the franchise, the problem would be primarily one of determining the nearest institution with the necessary capability and acceptability to the local population.

The really difficult problems would arise in multihospital urban areas where the location of the hospital, the residence of its outpatient population—primarily indigent or Medicaid—and the usually different residence of its inpatient population provide three separate and often hard to reconcile variables. The easiest approach, from a strict efficiency point of view, would be to divide the city into precisely defined geographic districts, with more or less equal populations, grouped around designated district hospitals. This is what the Swedes have done in Stockholm, effective January 1971.

Aside from the obvious difficulty of reconciling the residential areas of the inpatient and outpatient populations in a large American city, this approach appears too rigid and arbitrary for other reasons. There is not enough consumer free choice. It is true that the public school system works reasonably well on a district basis. But there is probably more opportunity for abuse, bureaucratic indifference or professional arrogance, in the health care field than in education. Even in education there have been some very thorny problems, not only in the South but in many Northern cities. In the health field, millions of poor people have just achieved some degree of free choice for the first time in their lives, thanks to Medicare, Medicaid, and the other new financing programs. They will almost certainly resist being locked into a new, overly structured system.

At the same time, it is essential that some geographic divisions be made as the basis for rationalization—specifically, for definition of the franchised hospital's responsibility. Robert M. Sigmond, Vice President, Albert Einstein Medical Center, and one of the nation's leading authorities on hospital planning, is working on the concept of the "community" as a "target area" rather than a "service area."[20] This is a complex idea, involving definition of the hospital's "index of relevance," the extent to which the hospital is now used by the population in a given geographic area, and its "index of commitment," the extent to which the hospital has committed its own staff time and other resources to persons living in this area. The concept seeks to provide a way of assuring a reasonable degree of choice to both providers and consumers within a context of defined responsibility. The "target area" is probably not the final solution to this dilemma. But it has advanced the level of discussion and deserves to be carefully studied.

3. **Internal organization of the hospital.** The *sine qua non* of effective community health services is institutional management. Individual idealism and dedication on the part of the individual physicians, administrators, trustees, nurses, and other professionals, important as they are, are not enough in this day of specialization, massive technology, and massive costs. Neither is it enough simply to pass new laws, appropriate new money, or even establish a franchise system. None of these factors can be meaningful unless, and until, translated into organized —that is, institutionalized—patient care. This is a job for management—the management of that institution designated to assume and to carry out responsibility for providing comprehensive care to the community.

The importance of stronger, more streamlined hospital management, just to carry out existing responsibilities, was pointed out in Chapter 3. The requirement in H.R.17550, that a provider institution wishing to participate in Medicare and Medicaid must have in effect an overall capital plan and a budget (Chapter 4), illustrates the importance attached by the federal government to internal managerial controls as an element in efficiency and cost containment. How much more will this be true if the hospital assumes the vastly greater responsibilities inherent in the community franchise!

The need for improved corporate structure has been increasingly noted in recent years. Progress is being made, through mergers, regional, denominational, and other types of joint management, and efforts at internal rationalization. But nothing like enough. The basic problem of divided authority between medical staff and lay administration not only remains unsolved but is apparently being exacerbated as "the battle for control of the hospital" gets hotter.

There are some grounds, however, for belief that this problem, like so many other social problems, will never actually be solved but will simply disappear as underlying technologic and economic trends become clearer. It is worth recalling that the battle over the "corporate practice of medicine" was never "solved"; it just became irrelevant as doctors, hospital administrators, and legislators alike came to realize the indispensability of the hospital and as physicians themselves found it useful to incorporate for tax purposes. The battle now is for control of that corporation. The long and bitter argument over "socialized medicine" is similar. The term is rarely heard any more. The issue now is over control of present and future public health care dollars (Chapters 4 and 8).

Fundamentally, what was at stake in all these issues was money and the control of certain facilities—for example, hospital beds—that affected the amount of money that could be earned. In the new affluent health care economy, wherein all doctors can make a good living and have more than enough work to do (Chapter 1), the issue of money becomes less important than regularizing and controlling work schedules and sharing, rather than adding to, one's responsibilities. Struggles for power between strong men within the hospital arena will probably never cease. Hopefully not, for out of such struggles often comes important progress. But in the franchised hospital of the future, with its defined patient population, its defined responsibilities, and its stabilized financing, the old struggle over an inadequate number of dollars and the beds to make them possible should become largely irrelevant.

Does this mean that more doctors will serve on boards of trustees? Probably. But with the board's work load greatly increased through the new community-wide responsibilities, it would appear that those doctors who wish to serve on hospital boards will have to be motivated primarily by a sense of community service rather than individual gain. The same would be true of nurses or other hospital personnel.

The terms of the franchise would undoubtedly include certain minimal requirements with respect to the board, the medical staff, and administration. Formulation of such requirements will obviously call for careful study—at both state and federal levels. The board of trustees, as the principal legal and policy-making body for the entire community's health care programs, will obviously have to be highly representative, well trained, dedicated and hard working. Formulas for assuring meaningful representation of all segments of the community will have to be devised. Requirements as to orientation, attendance at meetings, and length of service will be needed. Above all, every effort must be made to assure independence of judgment and moral integrity. Any board that acts simply as a rubber stamp, for the administrator, the medical staff, or the state, has no *raison d'etre* and deserves to be abolished.

Similarly, minimal requirements will be needed for medical staff organization. Such requirements are already being formulated in some state licensing laws and, even more importantly, in the courts.[21] Some hospital staffs are, even now, rewriting their bylaws to bring them more into line with current realities and to emphasize the new community responsibilities.[22]

Among the numerous problems of internal management that would require attention and, in many cases, reorganization, two merit special mention:

a. In order to pull together their hitherto scattered and generally inadequate ambulatory programs and other activities aimed primarily at low-income groups, some hospitals have recently established departments of community medicine. Although the responsibility of these units varies from institution to institution, they generally encompass the indigent clinics, the emergency room, and such of the following programs as the institution may have: neighborhood health center, family health program, nursing home affiliations, social service, home care program, narcotics control program, etc.

Some community-conscious hospital authorities are concerned about this development, fearing that it could lead to "tokenism" or segregation of this type of hospital activity from the mainstream of its work. This is a real danger. On the other hand, it does appear to provide a device for consolidating and upgrading the "stepchildren" activities and giving them more visibility, more prestige, and more money in the hospital hierarchy. It also provides a focus for encouraging and training responsible participation by leaders of the poor and other population groups that make most use of these services.[23]

b. Labor relations is another area where most hospitals have been weak both in terms of internal managerial controls and community relations. The growing impact of unionism, rising labor costs, and the crisis in community relations experienced by many urban hospitals all dictate renewed attention to this area. The importance attached by most American industries today to good labor relations, symbolized by the ubiquitous vice president for industrial relations, will probably have to be reflected in hospital management as well. This, in turn, will call for more mergers or joint management. A 75-bed hospital cannot afford, all by itself, a good vice president for industrial relations.

4. **The relationship of the hospital to other health care providers in the community.** Some form of compulsory affiliation to the franchised hospital should be required of all licensed providers in the community, both professional and institutional. Such affiliation could be made a condition of licensure. In return, the hospital governing body would, as noted, have to be made representative of, or at least responsive to, the entire provider community.

The problem of physician affiliation is especially important. In most communities, where the overwhelming majority of all practicing doctors are already hospital-affiliated, this would present no special problem, except that doctors with multiple affiliations would probably have to designate one primary affiliation. In New York City and a few other areas the problem would be very difficult and would probably require special arrangements. As a corollary of compulsory affiliation, the hospital would be required to define physician hospital privileges in a meaningful manner, involving graded privileges with respect to patient care, acceptance of peer review and discipline, continuing education, and, ultimately, computerized, hospital-based records.

If this were done, the problem of quality and utilization controls would be solvable by means of peer review and the issue of group versus solo practice would be much less acute than at present. Indeed, such a system could mean a new lease on life for solo practice—for that dwindling minority of doctors who prefer it.

Serious consideration should be given to the possibility of substituting institutional malpractice liability and insurance for the present individual liability and insurance which has become such a burden to many doctors, and is raising costs inordinately without any commensurate improvement in the quality of care.

In connection with compulsory hospital affiliation for doctors, the following statement by Ray E. Brown is especially interesting:

> I believe that sometime in the not too distant future the American Medical Association may "reorganize" so that the local component of organized medicine is not the county medical society, but the hospital medical staff. The hospital medical staff is the viable group that is functioning every day. Therefore the hospital should become the local site for organized medicine.[24]

5. **The role of regional or areawide bodies.** Considerable progress has been made during the past decade with voluntary regional or areawide planning. The

limits of voluntarism in this respect become daily more evident, however. The mushroom growth of the for-profit chains is the most recent proof. New York State has demonstrated that the many positive values of voluntary regional planning can be combined with state authority to provide a stronger, more effective planning mechanism. Even in New York, however, the planning responsibility is too limited, too focused on avoidance of unnecessary beds and expenditures, and not enough on the positive promotion of needed programs. Under the franchise system, the hospitals would need considerable assistance both in working out and maintaining relations with satellite institutions in their own communities and in working out and maintaining relations with neighboring providers in other communities. The regional planning bodies should be prepared to give this assistance.

In addition, these bodies should be prepared to assume their share of responsibility under the franchise system. Such a system could never work if all decisions were left to the state. In large states, at least, it would be an administrative nightmare. The decision-making responsibility must be decentralized. The following formula is not perfect but may at least be suggestive.

A reasonable number of areawide or regional bodies should be established in all states, utilizing, insofar as possible, existing "B" agencies set up under the federal-state Comprehensive Health Planning program, or other health care planning bodies. When a state adopted the franchise system the regional bodies would work with the existing hospitals in their regions in the effort to establish viable "communities" for each of them, and to issue interim franchises to be validated by the state. In the first instance, this effort might require as much as a year or two.

Thereafter, any hospital applying for a new franchise, for a change in its existing franchise, or for public funds for new construction, or any nursing home or other licensed facility applying for some change in its relation to a franchised hospital, would be entitled to an interim decision from the regional body within 60 days.

If dissatisfied with the interim decision, the institution would have another 60 days to appeal to the state. The state would have the same 60 days to intervene if it appeared necessary to protect the public interest. In the absence of either of these two events—an appeal by an affected party or intervention by the state—the regional body's interim decision would become final. The state would also be given a limited period of time to overrule the regional body's decision. If it failed to meet this timetable, the decision would become final.

It is probable that many, perhaps most, of the existing regional bodies would not welcome any such decision-making responsibilities. A somewhat similar issue has been raised in connection with the new cost effectiveness amendments in H.R. 17550. As noted in Chapter 4, one of these amendments proposes that reimbursement to Medicare and Medicaid providers for capital costs, such as depreciation and interest, would be withheld with respect to capital expenditures in excess of $100,000 that are inconsistent with state or regional plans (Section 221). Although the stated purpose of this proposal is to encourage health planning activities in the states, the Association of Areawide Health Planning Agencies is vigorously opposing that portion which involves approval or disapproval decisions on the part of the agencies.

Two major points are stressed: (1) Most of the bodies are still too new or otherwise unprepared for such a responsibility, and (2) the proposed increase in the agencies' legal or quasi-legal powers would reduce their "influential persuasiveness" and thus be counterproductive.[25]

The reluctance of the regional bodies to take on additional work and responsibility is understandable but not unique. The same reluctance is probably felt by most of the nation's hospital administrators, doctors, state and federal officials, in short, nearly all of us. Why the regional planning bodies, alone of all tax-supported institutions, should be permitted the luxury of advising and consulting (in the Medicare situation they do want to be consulted by HEW or the state agency) without having to accept the burden of decision making is not clear. In any case, it is a luxury the health care economy can no longer afford. The federal government and numerous state and voluntary bodies have been supporting areawide planning, in one form or another, for a decade. If, after all this time, most of the agencies are still incapable—for structural or other reasons—or unwilling to take on this type of responsibility, other means may have to be found to provide the needed planning and regulatory functions at the regional level.

6. **The role of the state.** Each state, within the limits of a set of minimal federal guidelines, would write its own community health services law, establishing requirements for a hospital franchise and for a license for other providers, the affiliation arrangements linking them together, and the machinery for implementation of the entire program.

The principal administrative unit, in most states, would probably be located in the health department, and might be called the division of community health services. Logically, all state units dealing with personal health services should be brought together in this new division—the Hill-Burton program, the institutional and professional licensing programs, the maternal and child health programs, rehabilitation, mental health, etc.

The state comprehensive health planning body, the "A" agency, should be required to think through its relationship to the new program and position itself accordingly. If it wishes to play a responsible role in the state's community health services program, it might become the advisory council for the new division. If it feels that is too restricted and wishes to try to coordinate all the state's health activities, including Medicaid, professional education, environmental services, and so forth, it should be located in the governor's office. Such decision, of course, cannot be made by the state alone, apart from the federal Comprehensive Health Planning program, but this too will probably require extensive revision.

In the new division of community health services, one of the principal sections would be that responsible for administering the hospital franchise and for maintaining the state's total network of community health services programs. In certain areas—for example, neurosurgery or open-heart surgery—one or two such facilities would probably be adequate for the entire state. The state unit would have to designate such statewide facilities. In some states—for example, New Jersey, New York, and Pennsylvania—the problem of interstate relations would be important and would probably require interstate compacts of some sort.

As already indicated, interim decisions on new franchises, renewals, major program alterations under existing franchises, and applications for capital grants or loans would all be made by the appropriate regional body and would become final within 60 days unless appealed by one of the affected parties or unless the state unit decided to intervene in the public interest. Thus, the state would be responsible for final decision of any contested case and for general surveillance of the whole program.

The state program would be financed partly by state funds, partly by federal. The latter would be contingent upon the state's acceptance of the minimal federal guidelines for the national community health services program.

7. **The role of the federal government.** In this four-level process of planning and regulation of community health services—community, regional, state, and national—the role of the federal government is both residual and primary: residual in that it has no operational responsibility in the state planning and regulatory system; primary in that the guidelines for the whole program should originate with Congress and the Department of Health, Education, and Welfare. Also, various federal carrot-and-stick combinations, including federal income tax exemption, eligibility for federal grants and loans, and participation in Medicare, Medicaid, and other funding programs, would be used to prod cooperation on the part of state governments and individual hospitals.

It is obviously a difficult and highly important role. Too heavy a hand would lead to revolt and noncooperation. Indecisive leadership, of the type associated with the Regional Medical Program and Comprehensive Health Planning, would be just as bad. Most important of all, the federal government has to know what it wants and then how to persuade the states and the voluntary institutions to cooperate.

Much has been said in recent years of the need for reorganization of the federal bureaucracy in the health care field. Senator Kennedy, Senator Ribicoff, Walter McNerney, the Secretary's Task Force on Medicaid and Related Programs, the National Commission on Community Health Services, the 37th American Assembly, and this author have been among those recommending creation of a top-level National Council of Health Advisors to help coordinate all federal health activities, to be located either in the Office of the President or the Office of the Secretary of Health, Education, and Welfare.

The Task Force (McNerney) devoted a substantial section of its report (Section II-C) to the need for improved management of federal health activities, including not only a National Council but a thoroughgoing restructuring of the top echelons of HEW. It also included a recommendation which has important bearing on the proposed franchise system:

> The operation of health service activities should be decentralized through contractual agreements with public and private agencies. The principal features of such agreements should be specification of desired outcomes, rather than specific methods of operation, and evaluation and information systems that can assess performance in terms of output or results.

The need for improved federal management becomes greater every day as costs rise and programs are piled on top of programs without any effort at real coordination. It will be even more urgent if some form of national health insurance, with all that implies in terms of new federal responsibilities, is adopted. Among the most difficult tasks that would face HEW and such a new council would be pulling together the myriad federal programs now involved in one way or another with community health services. Probably half could be eliminated altogether; the others must be made to work together.

NOTES

1. See, for example, American Hospital Association. Statement on the changing hospital and the American Hospital Association. *Hospitals, J.A.H.A.,* July 1, 1965, p. 35.

2. See, for example, Statement by the Catholic Hospital Association Board of Trustees concerning comprehensive health care. *Hosp. Progr.,* June 1968, p. 72 ff.

3. The President's Commission on Heart Disease, Cancer, and Stroke, *Report to the President,* Dec. 1964.

4. *Health is a Community Affair* (Cambridge, Mass.: Harvard University Press, 1967), p. 215.

5. Crosby, E. L., Hospitals as the center of the health care universe. *Hospitals, J.A.H.A.,* Jan. 1, 1970, p. 52.

6. Incoming President Mark Berke's inaugural address. *Hospitals, J.A.H.A.,* Mar. 16, 1970, p. 61.

7. Brown, R. E., Patients should call the hospital first. *Med. Econ.* May 12, 1969, pp. 79-82.

8. Sigmond, R. M., Will medical practice become more hospital-centered? *Med. Econ.* May 11, 1970, p. 121.

9. Lee, R. V. *Med. World News,* July 11, 1969. Also, *Hospitals, J.A.H.A.,* Jan. 16, 1970, p. 43.

10. For example, the 37th American Assembly, comprising 71 nationally recognized authorities in health care and related fields, recommended, as part of the evolving comprehensive health care system, "emphasis on restructuring the role of the hospital to assure that it play a positive leadership role in the rationalization of community and regional health services." *The Health of Americans,* Report of the 37th American Assembly (New York: Arden House, Apr. 1970), p. 6.

11. Letter to author, Oct. 21, 1969.

12. See Chapter 6, Note 12.

13. Miller, G., Director of Research in Medical Education, University of Illinois College of Medicine, Chicago. See, also, Grove, W., The Illinois plan. *J. Amer. Med. Assn.* Nov. 3, 1969, pp. 871-875. Also, Darley, W., The community hospital and the FP curriculum. *Hosp. Practice,* Aug. 1968, p. 88 ff.

14. For the story of one health department that is trying to exert leadership, see Ingraham, N. R. and Lear, W. J., A big city strives for relevance in its community health services. *Amer. J. Public Health,* May 1970, p. 804.

15. See, for example, the special issue of *Hospitals, J.A.H.A.,* on the plight of the public hospital, July 1, 1970.

16. Commonwealth of Massachusetts, Governor's Office, Press release, Apr. 14, 1970.

17. See, for example, Godber, G. E., The future place of the personal physician. Michael M. Davis Lecture, University of Chicago, 1969. Also, Somers, A. R., The hospital is the core of the system. *Mod. Hosp.,* Sept. 1970, pp. 87-91.

18. See, for example, Faltermayer, E. K., Better care at less cost without miracles. *Fortune,* Jan. 1970, pp. 81 ff.

19. The inevitable failure of complete *laissez-faire* in a world of limited resources has been eloquently argued by Garrett Hardin, a biologist at the University of California, Santa Barbara, in an article that has become a classic, The tragedy of the commons. *Science,* Dec. 13, 1968, pp. 1243-48. Excerpts from this article appear in Appendix A.

20. Albert Einstein Medical Center, *Planning Patterns,* Feb. 1970.

21. For a brief summary of court decisions affecting hospital medical staffs, as of mid-1969, see, Somers, A. R., *Hospital Regulation: The Dilemma of Public Policy* (Princeton University, 1969), pp. 21-27.

22. See, for example, Sigmond, R. M., The health care crisis and the planning process. Collected Papers from the Hospital Medical Staff Conference, University of Colorado School of Medicine, 1969.

23. For description of a successful program of community medicine undertaken by a large urban hospital, the Brooklyn-Cumberland Medical Center, and the organization and operation of the Fort Greene Community Medicine Board, its liaison with the community, see, Bergen, S. and Schatzki, M., New directions for an urban hospital, *J. Amer. Med. Assn.* (in press).

24. Brown, R. E., Changing management and corporate structure. *Hospitals, J.A.H.A.,* Jan. 1, 1970, p. 80. The following note suggests that Mr. Brown's prediction may be coming true: "Combine hospital staff and medical society meetings? That's what the Chicago Medical Society is thinking of doing to overcome poor attendance at meetings and to get doctors more involved in community needs. The plan calls for a doctor to designate a hospital where he attends staff meetings as the place where he'll also attend society meetings. Medical society business would be transacted during or following staff meetings." *Med. Econ.* July 20, 1970, p. 41.

25. *Comments on H.R. 17550,* Testimony prepared for the Senate Finance Committee, June 26, 1970 (mimeo).

Chapter 8

NATIONAL HEALTH INSURANCE: MAJOR PROPOSALS, ISSUES, AND GOALS

> The dilemma we are faced with is to bring millions of additional people under health insurance coverage which they urgently need without placing undue stress on our medical system, without encouraging prices to rise, and without creating further tensions among patients and taxpayers on the one hand, and physicians and hospital and health administrators on the other.
>
> WILBUR J. COHEN
> *Michael M. Davis Lecture* (1970)

Debate on the subject of national health insurance for the American people has ebbed and flowed for nearly 60 years.[1] On several occasions public opinion polls have indicated a small majority in favor of some such scheme.[2] Legislative proposals have been repeatedly introduced into Congress. As of October 1970, none had been voted out of committee. With the passage of Medicare in 1965, probably the majority of both proponents and opponents believed that the issue had been settled, at least for a decade or so.

The New Push for National Health Insurance

On the contrary, there is now stronger and more widespread support for some form of national health insurance than at any time in the past. The principal reasons are evident: the apparently uncontrollable rise in health costs—a rise that is threatening the viability of many of our major health care institutions as well as the access of many consumers to needed health services; the difficulties faced by many private health insurance carriers in maintaining the present level of benefits, let alone improving benefit coverage; the general popularity of Medicare; and the crisis in Medicaid and its implications for local, state, and even national politics.

Once again, as in the case of Medicare, labor led the way. The AFL-CIO has never altered its position in favor of national compulsory health insurance. It is currently (October 1970) supporting a bill (H.R.15779) introduced by Representative Martha Griffiths of Michigan in February 1970.

In February 1969, the United Automobile Workers, a union that has long played an aggressive and constructive role in the effort to expand both public and private health insurance, set up the Committee for National Health Insurance (CNHI),

[1]For this and succeeding notes in this chapter, see page 149.

headed by its respected president, Walter Reuther, later killed in a plane crash, and including such influential figures as Dr. Michael DeBakey, Mrs. Mary Lasker, Senators Edward Kennedy and John Sherman Cooper, and Whitney Young Jr. In July 1970 the Committee unveiled its "Health Security Program."[3] The following month, Senator Kennedy, together with 14 other senators, introduced S.4297 embodying the CNHI recommendations.

Governor Nelson Rockefeller, who has suffered more from the Medicaid confusion than any other governor, came out for a national insurance scheme early in 1969. Previously he had unsuccessfully urged compulsory health insurance for most employed persons in New York State. Prodded by Rockefeller, but clearly with an eye to their own growing welfare and Medicaid problems, the National Governors' Conference, meeting in Colorado Springs in September 1969, endorsed the general principle of national health insurance along with the recommendation that the federal government take over all welfare costs.

In April 1970, Senator Javits introduced his "National Health Insurance and Health Services Improvement Act of 1970" (S.3711). About the same time, the prestigious American Assembly recommended that "The nation should commit itself to a universal financing system for comprehensive health care, with public-private participation, generally referred to as national health insurance."[4]

Perhaps the most significant aspect of the current debate, however, is that this time the major provider organizations are not in opposition—at least not to the general idea. The AMA has been on record with its own brand of national health insurance, "Medicredit," since 1968.[5] In 1969 Representative Fulton of Tennessee and Senator Fannin of Arizona introduced companion bills comprising major features of Medicredit, and in July 1970 Representatives Fulton and Broyhill of Virginia introduced a new version, H.R.18567.

In September 1969, Dr. Edwin L. Crosby, Executive President of the AHA, announced that a Special Committee on Provision of Health Services (Perloff Committee) would undertake a study of national health insurance, along with related issues.[6] At the present writing, the Perloff Committee had not yet reported.*

In September 1969, Robert H. Finch, Secretary of Health, Education, and Welfare, instructed the McNerney Task Force on Medicaid and Related Programs (Chapter 4) to study the problem of "long-term methods of financing the Nation's medical care" and to develop recommendations. Even before the Task Force reported, however, Secretary Finch suggested—in response to Senate criticism that it had not considered the relationship between Medicaid and the proposed Family Assistance Plan (FAP)—a program of compulsory health insurance for all those who would receive aid under the family plan.

By the time the Task Force turned in its report, June 1970, Secretary Finch had departed from HEW and the new Secretary, Elliot Richardson, had arrived. As already noted, the Task Force made numerous recommendations, including one that the cost of the basic Medicaid benefits be completely federalized. On the question of national health insurance, however, it made no commitment, although some commentators are so interpreting its call for "a new national policy for health care

*As noted on page 109, the Committee's report on "Ameriplan" was published at the close of 1970.

financing." The Task Force urged the Secretary to appoint another high-level body "to undertake promptly a study directed toward development of a health care financing policy for the nation" and "to present recommendations to the Secretary in time for consideration during the 1971 session of the Congress."[7]

The Task Force's own contribution to the national debate was embodied in a set of "central and necessary objectives against which long-range financing proposals should be evaluated" and a long list of specific issues and questions, arising out of the previously stated objectives, which, the Task Force said, should be considered in evaluating all financing proposals. At the present writing, the proposed committee has not been appointed. And Undersecretary John G. Veneman's testimony during the brief Senate hearings on the Kennedy bill, September 23, 1970, indicated general opposition to compulsory national health insurance.[8]

Equally important, the House Ways and Means Committee, which claims the right to initiate all such legislation, a right that one or more Senate committees are threatening to challenge but without much hope of success, has given no indication that it is ready for any decisive action.

On the other hand, in order to get FAP—the welfare reform program—through Congress, the Administration is committed to submit a Medicaid replacement by 1971. This could represent the "opening wedge" for national health insurance or it could constitute a politically acceptable "cop-out" for the Administration.

In any case, the great debate over national health insurance is still far from its climax. Meanwhile, the time has come to move on from the usual litany of criticism of existing financing programs, public and private, and to make a serious effort to assess the probable results, both good and bad, of the various proposals that are being advanced. Under each, what is to be gained and what is to be lost? Are there more satisfactory paths to the same goals?

The rest of this chapter presents: (1) a summary of the major bills and proposals, as of October 1970, (2) a set of 10 goals or criteria by which these and the new bills, sure to be introduced in the 92nd Congress, may be evaluated, and (3) a brief attempt to evaluate the major proposals and to narrow the range of choice.

Three Broad Approaches

To begin with, it is essential to define what we mean by "national health insurance" by sorting out and classifying the major current proposals. Broadly speaking, there are three categories:[9]

  1. A federal program, with compulsory coverage of all or most of the civilian population, with broad and explicitly defined benefits, financed by a combination of payroll taxes and general federal tax revenues, and administered by the federal government without use of private carriers.

  2. A federal program of voluntary income-tax credits to taxpayers and vouchers to nontaxpayers, to help them purchase private health insurance, with minimal benefit standards, and financed entirely out of general revenues.

  3. Various in-between proposals embodying some characteristics of each of the above.

Category One: The Labor Proposals

There are two major proposals in Category One, both supported by organized labor: the Griffiths bill, sponsored primarily by the AFL-CIO, and the Kennedy bill, based on the CNHI Health Security Program. The two bills are basically similar.

Both aim for universal coverage. The Kennedy bill specifies that every resident of the United States will be covered. The Griffiths bill covers all citizens (except active-duty members of the uniformed services) and aliens who have been resident for at least a year or come from a country with reciprocal health benefits. The Kennedy proposal would terminate Medicare and the Federal Employees Program as well as the personal health components of the OEO, vocational rehabilitation, maternal and child health, and crippled childrens' programs. Medicaid and CHAMPUS (Civilian Health and Medical Program of the Uniformed Services) would continue as residual programs, providing such benefits as exceed the broad Health Security limits (see below). The Griffiths bill is silent on these points, but presumably it would have approximately the same effect. Private health insurance has no role in either bill.

With respect to benefits, both bills provide a broad range, including all necessary physicians' services and hospitalization. Both specify certain limits on most other services. For example, both limit initial dental benefits: Kennedy to children under 15 and exclusive of most orthodontia; Griffiths to children under 16 and others "who meet eligibility requirements for Medicaid or financial or other requirements set by the Board."

Outpatient psychiatric care is covered in full by Kennedy if provided in a hospital or by a comprehensive health service organization, community mental health center, or other approved institution. Private care is limited to 20 consultations during a spell of illness and inpatient care to 45 days per spell of illness. Griffiths appears to impose no limits in this respect. In the case of skilled nursing home care, Kennedy has a limit of 120 days per spell of illness; Griffiths, no limit. As to prescribed drugs, Griffiths is unlimited; Kennedy calls for a national formulary and, based on this formulary, unlimited coverage for inpatients and for persons enrolled in a comprehensive health service organization. For others, drug coverage applies only with respect to a list of chronic diseases and conditions requiring especially long or costly drug therapy.

The Griffiths bill's more liberal provisions with respect to several of the minor services is presumably balanced by a $2 copayment for each physician and dental visit after the first, and for home health services. Copayments are limited, however, to a yearly maximum of $50 per person, $100 for a family.

Both proposals would be financed on a tripartite basis from general federal tax revenues, employers, and employees and other individuals. The proportions coming from the three sources would be somewhat different. The CNHI proposal spoke in terms of 40 percent federal, 35 percent from employers, 25 percent from beneficiaries. Griffiths requires the federal contribution to equal three-fourths of the tax on employers and employees—43 percent of the total.

The tax rate specified in Griffiths is 3 percent of payroll for employers, one percent of wages for employees, and 4 percent of self-employment income. The Kennedy bill sets the initial rates at 3.5 percent on employers, 2.1 percent on employees. Instead of a tax on the self-employed, it proposes a 2.1 percent tax on all nonwage income over $400 and up to $15,000. Both bills propose raising the cut-off point for payroll taxes to $15,000. Both propose that funds be deposited in a special federal fund from which benefit payments would be made.

For programs of such magnitude, the administrative provisions of both bills are only sketchily developed. Both call for total operation by the federal government —HEW and its regional units. Private intermediaries are excluded, although Kennedy permits the delegation of the payment function to a regional medical society or other designated representative of a profession.

At the national level, Kennedy calls for a five-man full-time Health Security Board, appointed by the President and serving under the Secretary of Health, Education, and Welfare, to establish policy and regulations, and an executive director appointed by the board. The board would also be assisted by an advisory council, with consumers holding majority membership, and technical advisory committees. The Griffiths bill proposes a nine-man board, six full time, with three top HEW officials *ex officio*. This board would be advised by a consumer council and a professional council. Both programs provide that the national boards shall establish standards for participating providers.

In addition to the 10 regional HEW offices, Kennedy proposes establishment of a series of health service areas, which might or might not coincide with state lines. Both bills specify that each regional office (under Kennedy the area office, too) should have its own advisory council and technical committees.

The administrative philosophy behind the Kennedy bill—a nationwide health care budgeting system—was stated clearly in the CNHI report:

> Each year an advance determination will be made of the total amount to be spent in the various regions on physicians' services, institutional services, and other categories of services provided in local communities. The cost of each kind of service and the overall cost of the Health Security Program will be allowed to increase only on a controlled and predictable basis. . . .

> The size of the annual Health Security Trust Fund will be determined by the health insurance taxes and the federal government revenue contributions. . . . After an appropriate percentage of the Fund is set aside for contingency reserves and for the Resources Development Fund [see below] the remaining money will be divided among the ten regions, with regard for recent and current patterns of utilization of, and expenditures for, personal health services of the kinds covered by the program. In FY 1969 figures, this would have represented a national per capita allocation of approximately $200 (adding up to a total of $37 billion), but with higher and lower per capita amounts in the several regions.

Under this plan, institutional providers would be paid exclusively on an approved budget basis. Money for payment of physicians and other practitioners would be distributed to local areas within the region on a per capita basis with some adjustments. From the physicians' allotment, first priority would be given to those on salaries, those working in comprehensive organizations, and others agreeing to accept capitation payments for the care of a defined population. The remainder of the local fund available for physicians' services would be used for payment of fee-for-service physicians on the basis of fee schedules.

Quoting again from the CNHI report, "If the amount available for fee-for-service payments is in danger of being exceeded, payment of bills will be prorated." Providers would not be permitted to charge anything over and above the official fee. All payments would be made directly to providers; there would be no billing or indemnification of patients.

The Griffiths plan provides somewhat more flexibility with respect to payments. Hospitals could be paid on the basis of capitation, budgeted costs, or any other basis approved by the regional director "which shall provide incentives for improving the quality of care and the efficiency by which hospital services are delivered." With respect to practitioner services, the regional offices are expected to enter into capitation agreements with state or local medical societies, medical groups, or other nonprofit organizations. In turn, the latter may reimburse the individual practitioner on the basis of capitation, salary, fee-for-service, contract, or any combination thereof. An additional allowance of up to 5 percent would be made to participating organizations for innovations, including quality review, improving efficiency, and continuing education.

Both programs candidly aim to restructure the delivery system, especially to promote comprehensive health service organizations. Prior to the effective date of the Health Security Program, the Kennedy bill calls for a massive multimillion dollar planning and grant-in-aid program, aimed both at facilities and personnel training. After HSP became effective, there would be a separate Health Resources Development Account in the Trust Fund. A percentage of the fund's annual income, starting at 2 percent and rising to 5 percent, would be used for this purpose. The Griffiths bill also provides a revolving fund aimed at development of comprehensive delivery systems.

Category Two: The Tax-Credit Bills

Illustrative of the tax-credit approach is the Fulton-Broyhill bill, H.R.18567. Although more liberal than its 1969 predecessor, it is still at the opposite end of the spectrum from the labor proposals.

It is voluntary. Neither Medicare nor any other public health care program would be terminated, although presumably the Medicaid load would be reduced. The main purpose is to assist individuals and families to purchase private health insurance through a system of graduated federal income-tax credits or federally financed certificates in lieu of such credits.

The credits range from 98 percent of the total health insurance premiums paid for a 12-month period, if the tax liability is in the range of $301 to $325, down to 10 percent, if the tax is $1300 or more. Low-income families or individuals whose tax liability is zero or less than $300 would be eligible for a premium certificate to be used to buy health insurance from a private carrier. Income-tax payers could also opt for an insurance certificate if they prefer. The carrier would present the certificate to the federal government for redemption.

To qualify for the federal subsidy an insurance policy would have to provide (1) "basic benefits" consisting of (a) up to 60 days of inpatient hospital care, for which two days in an extended care facility could be substituted for one hospital day, (b) an unspecified amount of emergency room or hospital outpatient care, and (c) complete coverage of MD or DO services; and (2) one or more of the following "supplemental benefits": prescription drugs, additional inpatient days, blood in excess of three pints, major medical coverage up to $25,000, with a $300 corridor on top of the basic benefits, and one or more other personal health services provided under direction of a physician.

For all but the low-income beneficiaries, a $50 deductible for institutional care and 20 percent coinsurance on most other benefits are applicable. There are no dollar limits on the amount of allowable premium, but duplicate benefits are ruled out. States may buy in for Medicaid beneficiaries.

There are no special taxes to finance this program. It would be paid for entirely out of federal general revenues.

The administration is unclear. The premium certificates would be issued by the Secretary (presumably of HEW, although this is not explicitly stated). Presumably the Internal Revenue Service would monitor the tax-deduction provisions. State insurance departments would be responsible for approving insurance carriers and policies.

A Health Insurance Advisory Board of 11 persons, including the Secretary of HEW and the Commissioner of Internal Revenue, would be responsible for drawing up regulations, establishing standards for the states to follow in determining whether a carrier and a plan are qualified, and generally developing quality and utilization control programs.

A unique feature of the bill provides for establishment in each state of a peer review organization (PRO) to review "the need for and quality of . . . medical and other health services and the appropriateness of charges for such services." Each PRO would be established through agreement between the Secretary and a state medical society or organization designated by the society. If the society is unable or unwilling to enter into such an agreement, the Secretary could act on his own.

In any case, a PRO commission would be established in each state, consisting of five MDs or DOs, and the commission would appoint a number of local review panels, consisting of three MDs or DOs, for each part of the state. This network of local panels and state commissions, consisting entirely of physicians, would be responsible for passing on all questions relating to the reasonableness of charges, the quality of care, or the need for care, not only under the proposed new program but under existing Titles 5, 18, and 19.

Advisory councils, including representatives of consumers, providers, and carriers, would be appointed by the state medical society (at the state level) and by the commission (at the local level) to advise with respect to "administration and policy." Recommendations for professional discipline would be submitted by the commission to the Secretary for action. The latter, however, would be subject to court review.

Category Three: The "In-Betweens"

The bills and proposals that fall into this category are so diverse that a case could be made for listing each separately. However, the similarities are more important than the differences. All are between the extreme centralization of Category One and the extreme permissiveness of Category Two.

Although it is the most recent, the most fully developed proposal in this class is Senator Javits' bill, S.3711. It starts by improving Medicare and extending it to the entire population. The first step involves coverage of disabled social security beneficiaries and merger of Parts A and B—both financed through payroll taxes. The second step would cover all remaining citizens and some aliens. The benefits would be those of the present Medicare plus some drug and dental benefits and annual physical examinations.

Financing would be tripartite, but the federal share would be limited to that necessary to pay for the unemployed and public assistance recipients. Employers and employees would pay equal amounts, starting at 0.7 percent of the first $15,000 of wages or salary in the first year, up to 3.3 percent after four years.

Like Medicare, the new program would be administered by the Secretary of Health, Education, and Welfare, but below the federal level administration would be highly pluralistic, with numerous options. Private intermediaries would be continued, as under Medicare, except that in areas where no efficient private intermediary can be found, the Secretary is authorized to set up a federal health insurance corporation or to contract with a state for this purpose. Approved private carriers, under contract with HEW, may also sell plans that provide equivalent benefits at a cost equivalent to the national program. Employer-employee plans may also be continued provided their benefits are superior to the national program and the employer pays at least 75 percent of the cost.

No specific method is spelled out for payment of providers. The Secretary is instructed to study and promulgate a new reimbursement method by 1973. The new method "will be designed to control, and if possible reduce costs and utilization, to improve the organization and delivery of health services, yet assure that such control and improvement will not deprive providers or suppliers of care of 'fair and reasonable compensation'."

The Javits bill also encourages the development of more effective health care delivery systems, provides special grants for group practice plans, and authorizes contracts with "comprehensive service systems" on a basis that will enable them to share in any savings.

Governor Rockefeller was the first to sponsor legislation of this general type. Bills providing for statewide compulsory health insurance have been introduced, unsuccessfully, into the last four sessions of the New York State Legislature. In general, these bills have provided that all employees of firms with more than a specified number of workers (by 1970, it was down to one) must be covered by health insurance, to be paid for jointly by employer and employee. Minimum premium rates. as a percentage of payroll, and minimum benefit standards were specified, but the insurance could be purchased from any approved carrier. The government would contribute on behalf of low-income employee groups, the short-term unemployed, and welfare recipients.

J. Douglas Colman, President, Associated Hospital Service of New York, endorsed the Rockefeller approach in testimony before the New York Joint Legislative Committee on the Problems of Public Health. He recommended:

> . . . a legislative mandate of a minimum set of health care benefits as a condition of employment with the costs shared between the employee and the employer and with some form of underwriting from tax funds for low-income employees and fringe employers.[10]

With respect to benefits, Mr. Colman stressed the problem of reconciling the desirability of comprehensive coverage with existing manpower and other shortages and concluded:

> I think the legislative approach to universal health care must (1) start at expenditure and benefit levels not too far distant from those now widely in use, such as the Federal Employees Program, (2) emphasize universal coverage for substantially all gainfully employed people and their dependents, (3) encourage the use of the same benefit and delivery mechanisms for those not gainfully employed, and (4) be carefully designed to ensure the productive use of any new purchasing power it generates and prevent its dissipation in price rises or services that do not contribute to the health or welfare of the patient.

Ray E. Brown also appears to endorse the Rockefeller approach, although he uses the term "mandated insurance":

> People talk of compulsory health insurance, but that has a negative connotation. Somehow it says that the government is going to take over. I think that what we need is for the federal government to pass a law saying that every employer of one or more persons must carry a level of health benefits that is set by the federal government. . . . Then the third-party payers and insurance companies could fight it out as to who could deliver that package at the lowest price and who would retain the least out of it [in administrative overhead]. . . . In this way private enterprise or the private sector would competitively fight for the business. The third parties could not put in the small type or leave out benefits. . . . Unions could still negotiate for better benefits. It would put a floor under benefits without putting a ceiling on them.[11]

The most constructive proposal from the commercial insurance industry has come from Daniel W. Pettengill, Vice President, Aetna Life and Casualty, the company which has long administered the indemnity benefit plan of the Federal Employees Program on behalf of an industrywide consortium. Mr. Pettengill's plan is twofold: (1) federal standards for private group health insurance, enforced by means of reduced income-tax deductions from employers in case of noncompliance, and (2) federal promotion of "a uniform plan of health insurance benefits to the poor, near-poor, and uninsurable" by means of statewide "reinsurance pools" operated like a group, underwritten by all carriers in the state, administered by a single carrier, and with statutory benefit standards.[12] The "near-poor" and "uninsurables" would be required to pay something toward their insurance. Federal-state subsidies would make up the difference as well as the total cost for "the poor."

Speaking to a special meeting of the United Hospital Fund of New York, January 1970, this author suggested extension of a modified version of the Federal Employees Health Benefits Plan (FEP) to all the population not now covered by Medicare.[13]

What distinguishes this group of proposals from those in Category Two is the insistence on compulsory or "mandated" coverage, compulsory or required minimum benefits, financing through a combination of payroll taxes and general tax revenues, and an identifiable and accountable administration.[14] What distinguishes them from Category One is the continued use of private health insurance, in one form or another, and administrative decentralization.

Goals for an Acceptable Program of National Health Insurance

Before an overall comparison and evaluation of the various national health insurance proposals is attempted, it is essential to define a set of goals, or criteria, by which the different plans can be measured. One such yardstick was contained in the report of the Medicaid Task Force. The following 10 points utilize several of the Task Force concepts but depart from them in others. For more detailed study, the reader is referred to the Task Force's "Specific Issues for Investigation" in Appendix B.

1. **Universal coverage of the resident civilian population without distinction as to income or contributions.** Every vestige of the destructive and unadministrable means test, with its corollary two-class system of care, should be abolished. This does not mean that there should be complete uniformity of coverage. Different carriers—both public and private—are not only permissible, but desirable, provided consumers may choose among them on some meaningful informed basis and are not assigned on the basis of income.

2. **Comprehensive benefits.** This is another way of saying that the financial barrier to essential health care must be removed for all eligible participants. It does not mean that the program must necessarily cover every conceivable health service. It does not mean that patients should not contribute a penny toward their care.

It does mean that within the definition of comprehensive health care, given at the beginning of Chapter 7, the program should (1) aim to remove all financial obstacles to access to such care; (2) be reasonably certain that the benefits promised can actually be provided, that is, are not just "paper rights"; and (3) include a spectrum of services broad enough so that for the average patient something in the order of 75 percent of all health care would be "free" at the time of use.

The uncovered expenditures would be essentially of three types: (1) Small fees for physician and dentist visits and some drugs. Evidence from Kaiser and other programs that have used such fees does not indicate that they provide any real financial barrier. They can help to spread the total costs and also to discourage some unnecessary use of scarce resources. (2) Long-term care in mental hospitals or nursing homes. The question as to whether such care should be covered under the national insurance scheme or through some other public program can be argued both ways. In general it seems wise not to try to concentrate every type of public health responsibility into the single insurance program. The result is likely to be a reduction in total available funding. If this is not done, however, it means that some fairly sizable portion of the population will have medical needs well beyond those available through the insurance scheme, thus requiring a residual Medicaid-type program. (3) A certain amount of care that is desirable from the point of view of the individual but not essential from the point of view of society, for example, contact lenses, cosmetic surgery, and some teen-age orthodontia.

3. **Pluralistic and competitive underwriting.** Expansion and improvement of Medicare, as the core of the national health insurance system, is desirable both as a means of assuring coverage for all who find it difficult to obtain private insurance and as a competitive yardstick for evaluation of the private programs.

Competitive underwriting by a limited number of private carriers, along the lines of FEP, should provide many advantages, including a brake on bureaucracy and/or political interference, and a way of encouraging innovation in both quality and cost controls. By providing a limit on the number of carriers permitted to compete under the national scheme, it should be possible to achieve a good compromise between unlimited competition, which has clearly proved unsatisfactory in the health insurance field, and monolithic government operation.

4. **Consumer free choice as far as practical.** The term "free choice" has been so much abused, in the past, as a propaganda slogan in the war against health insurance and third-party programs of all types that, for many, it has lost all meaning. Actually, the concept is as important as democracy or political freedom. People who are denied all choice in health care are not likely to develop a responsible attitude toward the use or abuse of that care or even their own health. Free choice is an important factor in health education and health maintenance.

Needless to say, it has to be reconciled with essential quality controls. People cannot claim the right to use quacks or to pursue illusory cancer cures at public expense. Even here, the boundaries are never clear-cut. In general, all persons, no matter how poor, should have the right to at least two *informed* options as to the type or system of health care they prefer. (The uninformed "free choice" available to the middle class in some communities today is often less meaningful than the informed choice available to FEP members, for example.) This means that even the very poor should not be "districted" or "locked into" a single source of primary care because it is the only one covered by the insurance program.

5. **Adequate and stable income for providers.** In the effort to remove the long-standing financial barrier suffered by many patients in the past, it would be shortsighted to attempt to impose unreasonable restrictions on the income of providers. The word "attempt" is used because in so rich a country it probably would not be successful. Given the present supply and demand imbalance, many providers would find ways of operating outside the system.

Moreover, such restrictions are unnecessary. Punitive motives have no place in a financing mechanism, whether one is thinking of unreasonable doctors or irresponsible patients. This nation can afford to pay its health care providers adequately and should do so. Of course, the definition of "adequate," like the definition of "reasonable" under Medicare, is subject to many interpretations. It is just as foolish, from the point of view of the providers as well as the public, to build inflation into the payment system as to try to use it to deflate.

The question of stability is particularly important. One of the major shortcomings of Medicaid from the providers' point of view is the uncertainty of payment—both the amount and the timing. Providers cannot be expected to operate in a responsible manner unless the government, soon to be the principal source of income for most, sets a correct example. The vagaries of legislative appropriations, especially at the state level, are particularly demoralizing.

The impact of health insurance on the capital costs of institutional providers, on capital financing, and on the money market in general is, as noted earlier, beyond the scope of this book. In general it should be clear that the insurance scheme should not be permitted to inhibit normal capital expansion any more than it should be permitted to cause inflation in capital costs and the costs of obtaining money. Use of the payment formula to provide a portion of approved capital costs appears a sensible way of spreading such costs. Government grants and loans and private philanthropy will not only continue to be needed but also provide a useful means of diversifying the sources of needed funds.

6. **Incentives for efficiency and economy.** The kind of health care and health care system desired by most American consumers as well as providers will not be cheap. There is every reason to anticipate a continuing rise in national expenditures for this purpose, both absolutely and as a percentage of the GNP. Any national insurance program that is used as an instrument for rationing inadequate health care expenditures will be resented and circumvented. As in other areas of national life, Americans are prepared to tolerate a degree of duplication and waste in return for greater freedom. Thus far, we have felt this "margin for error" has paid off.

A rise in the proportion of GNP going for health care on the order of one percentage point every 10 years—more than in the 1950s, less than in the 1960s (Table 1)—is probably not unreasonable for the next two or three decades. Assuming only minimal inflation and population growth, this would probably be necessary just to allow for new cures, further advances in technology, and the greater demand that will inevitably accompany further improvement in life expectancy. Such expansion would bring us to about 10 percent of GNP by the year 2000.

On the other hand, freedom can degenerate into anarchy, and too generous funding can lead merely to inflation, which in turn can adversely affect quality. As noted in Chapter 4, we have seen private health insurance come close to destroying itself through lack of adequate regulation. We have seen Medicare and Medicaid threatened by uncontrolled inflation. Now that wages and salaries in the health care industry have nearly caught up with those in the general economy, there is little justification for the continued discrepancy in the price rise in this industry as opposed to the general cost of living. (With physicians' salaries so much out of line with those of nurses and other health care personnel, there may be some need for internal redistribution.) At this point the necessity for building some cost restraints into any proposed national health insurance scheme is essential. Similarly, all aspects of the program should be designed with considerations of efficiency in mind.

In designing incentives for efficiency, however, long-run considerations are as important as short-run. It probably seemed efficient, 25 years ago, to concentrate most of our health care resources in the hospital. The shortcomings of this approach are now apparent. It may now seem to some more efficient to ignore the hospital and concentrate resources in primary care units. This would merely reverse the error. Again what is needed is balance.

It is the same with methods of payment. Fee-for-service seemed not only normal but efficient in the past. Today, it is fashionable to lay heavy emphasis on capitation. The truth is that both methods have their advantages and disadvantages, as does salaried practice.

The British, who use a modified form of capitation for their general practitioners, have never used it for specialist care. In Sweden, where health care is also "socialized," no doctors are paid on the basis of capitation. There is much to be said for capitation, especially in a country where overdoctoring is as real a danger as it is with us. But it is not a panacea. To seek to impose it universally, as an efficiency and economy measure, would be self-defeating.

One technique of provider payment where the disincentives for efficiency are now abundantly clear is open-ended individual cost reimbursement for hospitals and other institutions. An alternative, acceptable to both the hospitals and the third parties, private or public, is so important as to be a prerequisite to a viable national health insurance scheme.

Incentives for economy should also be directed at consumers—one reason for small charges on practitioner services and some drugs and for consumer participation in the basic financing.

7. **Equitable financing.** From the point of view of both the family and the nation, the method of raising funds for national health insurance is as important as the total amount to be raised. Whether financed through general revenues, payroll taxes, income-tax credits, vouchers, out-of-pocket deductibles and coinsurance, or any combination thereof, the impact of a program of this magnitude (we are talking of something in the order of at least $50 billion if we aim for three-fourths of $64 billion, and it will be more each year) will inevitably be enormous.

The argument over "regressive" payroll taxes versus "progressive" income taxes —the major source of general federal revenues—is heated and real. The burden on some individuals of having to make cash payments, however small, at the time of illness has been criticized not only as inequitable but as a deterrent to preventive care. The income-tax credit device has been criticized as of no value to the poor and the voucher described as a thoroughly unreliable way of channeling needed care to this group.

Some of these methods appear to rule themselves out as inconsistent with the other goals of the program—universal coverage and comprehensive benefits. Some mix of general revenues, payroll taxes, and direct patient payment appears most equitable as well as productive of the necessary funds. Careful studies should be made of the probable effect of varying the proportions in this important recipe.

8. **Administrative feasibility.** No program can be better than its administration. The more ambitious, the more grandiose the scheme, the more complex its administration inevitably becomes. In a country of this size, with such marked regional, political, economic, and cultural variations, administration is inevitably difficult. And in an area as diffuse and intensely personal as health care, it is doubly so. As John Gardner, former Secretary of HEW, said, "Any organization setting out to cure social ills had better be sure it isn't creating problems as rapidly as it cures them."

In the first place, there is the temptation to do too little or too much. Some programs seem attractive precisely because they appear to require virtually no administration, to be almost self-administering. This usually turns out to be a costly fallacy. Workmen's compensation, for example, a program of "mandated" insurance coverage for injured employees, appeared to call for minimal administration. The self-interest of employers in keeping down their experience-rated premiums and the self-interest of workers in not getting hurt on the job, and the "no fault" payment of specified cash and medical benefits in case of an accident, all seemed to add up to a foolproof system wherein little administrative surveillance was needed.

In point of fact, the results of a half century of experience with workmen's compensation have been unsatisfactory. On the average, over the years, only about 55 percent of the amount that employers pay in premiums has been paid out in benefits, and of this 55 percent a substantial amount has been diverted into litigation costs.[15] In place of orderly benefit administration, there has been a never-ending battle between employers trying to hold down their premiums and injured employees trying to get more from the kitty.

At the other extreme, there is the possibility of too much or too highly centralized administration. This raises, again, the question of the public-private interface. The desirability of competitive private underwriting of a substantial portion of the population has already been indicated.

Should there, in addition, be private intermediaries for the core program? Arguments can be made pro and con. The "pro" argument is simply a variation on the argument for private underwriters: more competition should lead to more efficiency. However, it is clear that this argument can be pushed too far. It may not be possible for the same carriers to act as intermediaries for the government program at the same time that they are competing with that program, without creating an impossible conflict of interest.

9. **General acceptability to consumers and providers.** Any new method of financing health care must be acceptable both to the general public and to all categories of health care personnel and institutions. A system that continues to be resented by the major providers of care would be hampered by lack of cooperation and an inadequate long-run supply of doctors and other personnel. Similarly, it must be seen by most consumers as financially and administratively equitable and consistent with the cultural norms of the community.

The probability that the legislative debates over national health insurance will be dominated by the AMA on the one hand, and by organized labor on the other (the latter is now split into two factions, with the United Automobile Workers outside the AFL-CIO, but on health insurance at least there are no significant differences), should not be permitted to overshadow the vast majority of both providers and consumers who are outside these two political powerhouses. However, the extent to which these "middle Americans" find their concerns reflected in the evolving program will depend on the extent to which they take the trouble to make themselves heard.

10. **Flexibility in the face of changing supply and demand factors.** Health care is a highly dynamic area. Change is the only certainty. Any financing system that is totally in harmony with the underlying delivery system today will, almost certainly, be out of key tomorrow or at least the day after tomorrow. Provision for periodic revision, without having to go back to Congress each time, must be built into the new program. This means rather wide administrative discretion. It also means a certain looseness in administrative arrangements. There must be channels for ideas and innovations to flow up from the grass roots as well as downward from the leadership.

Moreover, it should be recognized that health care is not the only factor involved in health. Education, housing, pollution, and other factors play a significant, perhaps even more essential, role. The national insurance program should neither freeze expenditures at current levels nor lead to excessive future investment in health services. The way must be left open for the public to change its priorities.

Narrowing the Range of Choice: The Vital Center

It is beyond the scope of this book to attempt solutions to the dilemma of national health insurance in the United States. The aim is to clarify the major problems involved in the development of a viable national insurance system for this huge country, to delineate the desirable goals of such a system, and to establish guidelines for evaluation of the proposals that have been made and others that are sure to follow. In so doing, it should at least be possible to narrow the range of choice.

No effort will be made to compare the different proposals on the basis of estimated costs. In the first place, no reliable estimates are or can be available. The particulars of all the proposals are still in flux, and any estimate at this stage is inevitably ephemeral. Moreover, the experience of Medicare, where the most careful actuarial projections fell so far short of the mark, suggests that any evaluation keyed primarily to the dollar sign is likely to be misleading. The Administration's criticism of the Kennedy bill on the basis that it would cost $77 billion in the first year of operation was probably as conjectural as Leonard Woodcock's contention that this figure was $20 billion too high.[16]

Second, what really matters from an economic point of view is not the gross cost of any specific new program but the net cost—that is, what it adds to the nation's total health care expenditures. Thus the net cost of a program which absorbed Medicare would, in 1970, be at least $7 billion less than its gross. Similarly, the extent to which it absorbed Medicaid or other public programs would have to be taken into account.

Third, with respect to social utility, it is not the dollar cost of the program that is vital but the degree of protection, in terms of actual coverage of family health care costs, that those dollars would buy.

This discussion is aimed primarily at social value and workability—the basic factors underlying the 10 criteria discussed in the previous section. Measured by this yardstick, the Fulton-Broyhill version of Medicredit must be faulted on the majority of the 10 points. It offers no chance of approaching universality of coverage. Income-tax payers who do not participate would be penalized by losing their potential tax credits, but that is not the same thing as mandatory coverage. There is no penalty on the poor who do not take advantage of the government vouchers.

Consider this possibility. Vouchers are issued to millions of poor people who, for one reason or another, do not use them; or if they do, the insurance they buy is inadequate. They get sick and need help. What happens? Medicaid would obviously have to be continued as a major, rather than a residual, program.

Medicredit's major shortcoming, however, relates to the lack of administrative controls. Peer review of the quality and use of health services can be a valuable asset to both providers and consumers if carried on in a context of public accountability—for example, in a franchised hospital (Chapter 7). But the idea of substituting peer review, by five doctors appointed by a state medical society, for public administrative controls is so unrealistic that it is hard to believe it was seriously proposed.

Totally lacking in effective controls of any sort, the Fulton-Broyhill bill makes no contribution to increased efficiency and economy but would, almost surely, result in the reverse. If we have learned anything from the bitter experience of the past two decades, it is that simply pumping x billions of dollars into an already imbalanced supply-demand situation, without any administrative controls, does not buy better benefits. It buys only more inflation.

Since it subsidizes existing inappropriate patterns of coverage, it would run counter to new organizational trends which seek to encourage more primary care. And, ironically, since the results are so thoroughly unpredictable, it would provide little financial relief to the hospitals or any other hard-pressed providers. On the contrary, it would contribute to the general fiscal instability which is the source of so much of the present difficulty throughout the industry.

Since funding is entirely out of general federal revenues, the impact is not regressive, as it would be if totally funded out of payroll taxes. But, by the same token, the funding is probably less stable and less immune to political pressures of one type or another than if based, at least partly, on payroll taxes and administered through a trust fund.

The chief pluses to be cited for this proposal are: (1) It does not interfere with free choice for those who now have a choice; (2) it would offer some measure of relief to middle-class families, especially the self-employed who pay all of their own insurance premiums; and (3) it would at least establish the principle of federal regulation of health insurance. Some years ago, these might have been real contributions. Today, they are conspicuously too little and too late.

This is obviously not the only possible version of Medicredit. It is already better than the 1969 Fulton-Fannin bills. This process of liberalization can and probably will continue in the effort to win more public support. But it does not touch the basic flaw in the Medicredit approach. It is simply not possible, in the present condition of the health care economy, to provide anything like universal coverage, comprehensive benefits, and stable provider income without an effective administrative control mechanism. The income-tax-voucher combination is an ingenious effort to circumvent this basic fact, but it cannot succeed and, if tried, the results will, almost surely, do more harm than good.

The labor proposals are better bills. They aim to provide something approaching comprehensive coverage to nearly all Americans and at the same time to do something about the basic dysfunctions in the health care economy and the rampant inflation. Nevertheless, when rated against the 10-point yardstick, they, too, must be faulted on the majority of points. Their universality and comprehensiveness are self-evident. The claim to universality is particularly true of the Kennedy bill, whose sponsors flatly state their intention of replacing nearly all existing financing programs.

This is the opposite fallacy from Medicredit. Whereas the latter is too limited, this is too broad and all-encompassing. Whereas Medicredit makes no effort to correct, indeed underwrites, existing shortcomings of the private health insurance system, the labor bills tend to throw out the good with the bad. Private health insurance has, as noted in Chapter 4, many achievements to its credit. There are many excellent programs of various types—for example, FEP, Kaiser, GHI, San Joaquin, some of the Blue Cross programs, and some of the insurance company programs. Medicare not only has an impressive record of satisfied customers but, over a painful five-year period, has built up a body of administrative expertise probably second to none in the health insurance world. To think of dismantling most of these programs overnight without the assurance of anything better to put in their place except a well-motivated dream of universality and comprehensiveness is unwise and potentially dangerous.

In other respects, too, the labor bills provide a sort of mirror image of the Medicredit faults. Whereas Medicredit is at great pains to try not to interfere with the existing delivery system, the Kennedy and Griffiths proposals, especially the former, quite candidly seek to restructure the system, primarily toward prepaid group practice. The short shrift given to fee-for-service doctors with respect to payment and the discrimination against patients of fee-for-service doctors in respect to drugs are illustrative. This effort to manipulate both providers and consumers into a form of health care which, regardless of its appeal to the experts, is still distinctly a minority pattern is as unacceptable in a democracy as the AMA's traditional effort to straitjacket everyone into the fee-for-service system.

With respect to hospitals, Kennedy provides only one method of payment—approved budgets. Again, this is as bad as the Medicredit approach, which simply ignores the problem of effective controls over provider payments.

The administrative structure of both labor proposals appears, on the surface, as if it weren't meant to be taken seriously. Here are proposals that would inevitably involve well over $50 billion a year if their goals of universality and near-comprehensiveness are to be achieved. Some 200 million consumer-patients would be almost totally dependent upon the program for services of life-and-death importance. Most providers—some 300,000 physicians, and perhaps three million additional health workers, over 7000 hospitals, 20,000 long-term care institutions, and probably thousands of other health care facilities and programs—would be dependent upon the program for their income.

Yet it is proposed that a program of this magnitude, dealing in an area of such complexity, sensitivity, and controversy, should be administered out of one federal and 10 regional offices. Kennedy indicates the need for additional area offices, with ill-defined duties, but it is the one national board that would be responsible for reviewing and approving, *every year*, the budgets of *all* institutional providers as the *only* basis for their payment! This is as patently unsatisfactory as Medicredit's "no administration" proposal.

On one point, however, the two approaches appear to be in some sort of agreement—the downgraded role of the hospital. Both Kennedy and Griffiths rightly seek to promote more primary and ambulatory care. But in doing so they would build up power centers outside the hospitals. This could result in driving a new wedge between hospitals and doctors, and thus lead to further fractionation of the community health care system and impede development of the desperately needed integrated institutional responsibility for community-wide comprehensive care, the subject discussed in Chapter 7.

The extent to which Kennedy's Resources Development Account would displace Hill-Burton and other current sources of capital funds is not indicated, but a fundamental shift in priorities clearly is. The Fulton-Broyhill proposals for peer review and cost controls to be delegated to the medical societies would probably represent a further breakup of existing hospital controls without any assurance of equal effectiveness.

Finally, the labor bills are overly rigid, would almost certainly affect adversely the income of many providers, would probably interfere in some cases with consumer free choice, and while appearing to offer incentives to efficiency and economy in the short run would probably have the opposite result in the long run.

The chief merit of these bills, aside from the well-motivated concern with universality and comprehensiveness, is their financing. The progressive-regressive tax argument has been nicely resolved through tripartite funding. The small differences in the government proportions and in the employer/employee proportions need not be argued here. The Kennedy proposal is easier on the self-employed, more ingenious in its approach to nonwage income. On the other hand, the Griffiths bill is to be commended for its $2 physicians' visit fee—another way of spreading the cost. The logic of imposing this on home care visits is less evident.

All in all, however, it appears that these bills are also unacceptable in their present form. Whereas Medicredit was much too limited, these are too heavy-handed. Ironically, both would probably be self-defeating even in terms of their own avowed aims. The inflation and confusion likely to result from Medicredit would, almost certainly, lead to more stringent government controls than would be necessary if moderate controls were applied now. On the other hand, the monolithic labor bills would, almost certainly, lead to a large amount of health care being sought and being given totally outside the system and its controls. Since the ability to opt out of the system is, in practice, more readily available to the rich than to the poor, we could move again to a two-class situation. But this time the resulting political furor would be far more bitter. In short, while the labor sponsors aim for innovation and change in the delivery system, they have not yet designed machinery that appears promising for these objectives.

Just as the Fulton-Broyhill bill will not be the last word on Medicredit, we may anticipate numerous revisions of the labor proposals—what may be called for lack of a better phrase "the unitary approach." To begin with, there will probably be a consolidation of the Griffiths and Kennedy proposals and any others that follow the same general line. Then, as the new version is ground through the legislative mill, it will probably become more limited and less global, less restrictive and more flexible. There is obviously a great deal of room for negotiation and compromise in these proposals. Perhaps that was the mood in which they were presented.

This may be true of the AMA proposals as well. Perhaps we are witnessing a classic example of collective bargaining on a national scale. There is much to be said for the bargaining approach to resolution of difficult social problems. That is all the more reason to focus major attention not on the extremes, which are certain to be modified, but on the vital center—the middle of the road, where the acceptable compromise is almost sure to emerge.

So we turn to the four major proposals in this broad center area. A decade ago, the two-pronged Pettengill proposal, with its call for federal standards for private health insurance combined with publicly subsidized state reinsurance pools to enable private insurance to care for the indigent and medically indigent, might have saved the day for private insurance. It might have averted the need for Medicaid as well as national health insurance. Today it, too, is too little and too late. Medicare exists. So does Medicaid. Medical care costs are over 100 percent higher than they were 10 years ago; hospital costs nearly 300 percent.

There are, also, some basic shortcomings. Administratively, it might prove almost as impossibly difficult as the Fulton bill. Who would police all the hundreds of private carriers to make sure they lived up to the federal standards? If the standards were high enough to guarantee really comprehensive benefits to the nonpoor, could such policies be sold on a voluntary basis and without government subsidy?

The Rockefeller proposal for compulsory coverage through private insurance seeks to deal with some of the weaknesses of the previous plan. Coverage of most of the employed and their dependents is compulsory. Employers and most employees are required to make specified minimal payments. A new agency, the New York State Health Insurance Corporation, would receive broad administrative powers.

However, the New York bill excludes from compulsory coverage precisely those groups that most need it—the long-term unemployed, part-time employees, persons on welfare, and the self-employed. Protection could be purchased, on a voluntary basis and in different ways, for most of the excluded—for example, by the state for Medicaid patients—but that is far from universal coverage.

Furthermore, administration would still be extremely difficult. Few states have the administrative resources of New York and there is little reason to expect better performance with health insurance, in most of the 50 jurisdictions, than they have exhibited with workmen's compensation or unemployment insurance. The same forces of interstate financial competition within industry would work against raising benefits or broadening eligibility.

The most attractive aspect of the Rockefeller proposal is the attempt to combine strong public supervisory authority with private underwriting. However, if this goal is to be effectively achieved, the most promising approach would be to limit the number of carriers permitted to participate. And if this were done, we would, in effect, have made the step between mandated insurance and FEP's "controlled competition." Here, finally, in this area—which includes the Somers proposal for improvement and extension of FEP to the entire population, and the Javits proposal for improvement and extension of Medicare to the entire population with the additional option of private insurance if it meets the benefit and price standards of the public program—there lies the greatest hope for meeting all or most of the 10 criteria for solving the dilemma of health insurance posed by Wilbur Cohen (page 127).

The Javits proposal is, of course, the more fully developed. It reflects a great deal of sophisticated thinking and effort. It rates high scores on most of the 10 criteria. It is particularly ingenious in combining comprehensiveness of benefits with flexibility of administration, in combining a gradualistic approach with a not-too-distant timetable for full coverage, in offering something for everybody and a minimum of offense to anyone. It is pragmatic in that it builds on a going program and its administrative expertise. It is idealistic in that it looks toward universality and comprehensiveness.

Of course, it finesses one of the toughest issues, provider payment, by leaving that up to a new HEW study. Its principal weakness, however, is in the overly generous number of options, which could turn out to be almost as difficult to monitor as mandated insurance. Thus, the difficulty of reviewing and passing on every policy in the nation that claims to be as good as the improved Medicare would in itself be formidable. Then there is the same question we have asked with so many of the other plans: What happens to the individual who buys a pig in a poke? Who picks up the pieces?

By contrast with this carefully developed bill, the proposal to use the Federal Employees' Program as a model for a universal program is still only an idea. There are, however, many advantages in the FEP approach. Suitably modified to take into account the vastly larger and more heterogeneous population involved in a national undertaking, such a program could be molded to meet all the 10 criteria.

What would such a national health insurance program look like? There are many possibilities that should be explored. But here, for the sake of illustration, is one model.

The entire resident civilian population is covered on a compulsory basis and is eligible for benefits without regard to income or contributions. There is a single federal fund-raising mechanism, which has no relation to eligibility. The necessary funds are derived from four sources—federal general revenues, payroll taxes, tax on individual nonwage income, and direct patient payments.

Benefits are underwritten by a variety of insurers, including an expanded Medicare—the core program, which is available to the entire population—and a limited number of private carriers or carrier-consortia. Families and unattached individuals choose among these various carriers at periodic intervals, perhaps every two years.

The expanded Medicare benefit package constitutes the national minimum standard. But, within specified limits, other participating carriers design their own benefit packages.

Revenues funnel through a national health insurance trust fund which makes equal periodic capitation payments to Medicare and all the other participating carriers. The carriers, in turn, pay the providers. Presumably, by this time, Medicare will have established more rigorous reimbursement procedures and cost controls, which constitute a yardstick for evaluating all provider costs. However, the competing carriers are encouraged to work out alternative mutually-acceptable payment procedures with their providers. Economies resulting from such competition are shared by the carriers and the program as a whole.

The new program does not impose organizational change on the delivery system. For example, it does not discriminate against either fee-for-service or capitation. It is designed to allow change to develop freely in response to new technology, changing consumer needs and demands, and competitive experimentation. Moreover, it is highly flexible.

If, for example, it should turn out that private carriers, operating under an FEP-type program, are unable to exert effective cost pressures on providers and the necessary adjustments in delivery are not forthcoming, the decision is not irrevocable. Private underwriting could be terminated—a potent argument for maintaining Medicare as the core of the system—and the voluntary programs assimilated into a governmental program far more easily than the reverse. In short, such an approach provides maximum flexibility and maneuverability to enable the nation to meet future developments without giving irretrievable hostages to fate.

If its present attitude holds, organized labor would oppose the use of private carriers but, under these highly regulated conditions, their opposition might be altered. In any case, despite their great contribution, they cannot be permitted to hold a veto over a program that is designed for the entire nation, any more than can the AMA.

It is often forgotten that spokesmen for the Kaiser plan urged the FEP approach in 1965, when Medicare was being debated. For example, Dr. Clifford Keene, now President, Kaiser Foundation Health Plan, urging that the proposed bill be amended along FEP lines, stated:

> From the viewpoint of promoting sound public policy, the advantages of this approach are substantial. It will effectively implement the concept of significant choices which are fundamental in our society. It will preserve the opportunity for variation and experimentation on which continuing improvements in the organization of health care services depend. It will permit different kinds of health plans to continue covering their aged members, and it will permit direct service plans to continue doing this in a manner which stresses quality medical care under a system with built-in incentives for controlling costs.[17]

The relationship between this type of plan and the rationalized delivery system recommended in Chapter 7 was suggested in the model of Mercy Hospital, with its various sources of funds and its varied methods of paying providers. The key to success in such a pluralistic system is twofold: controlled competition and supervised free choice. Through a merger of elements of the Javits bill and the FEP model it should be possible to achieve this goal.

Even assuming agreement on the desirability of this general middle-of-the-road approach, a great deal more study will be needed. Many specific issues remain to be hammered out: the relation of the new program to Medicare; the manner and rate at which it would assimilate (or not assimilate) other public and private programs; benefit levels, premium rates, and the actuarial computations that tie them together; the precise technique for exercise of consumer choice; the administrative setup, complex in any case; and so forth. Better to take a little longer making the decision than to stumble into another half-baked plan as we did with Medicaid.

On the other hand, we cannot wait too long. There is real urgency, a financial crisis that threatens the lives and well-being of many Americans as well as the viability of important segments of the health care economy. To say that a plan is not "perfect" is no excuse for inaction. We shall never achieve a "perfect" plan just by studying it or talking about it. We have to start moving. Wilbur Cohen, one of the principal architects of Medicare, has suggested a realistic timetable:

> If we take the steps we can take now, we could have a comprehensive national health plan ready to begin operations in 1976, when we commemorate the 200th anniversary of the Declaration of Independence.[18]

Even in the years before the passage of such a law, the debate over such a pluralistic, competitive program should be conducive to greater experimentation with improved methods of delivery as well as new techniques of voluntary insurance, while anticipation of a single monolithic program would probably contribute further to a sense of fatalism with respect to voluntary methods and cost controls.

Conversely, enactment of a primarily political, stop-gap program such as the Administration is reported to be preparing for 1971—involving a federalized but separate program for the indigent or the proposed Family Assistance population, and a souped-up private insurance plan for the middle class—would not only perpetuate, but almost certainly exacerbate, some of the worst features of our present financing methods. The dishonored doctrine of "separate but equal" would acquire new meaning and cause new difficulties. Fragmentation would be intensified. The growing appreciation of the importance of comprehensive care and the slow but unmistakable trend toward a more efficient delivery system and more responsible, cost-conscious consumers and providers would be reversed. The effort to preserve a predominantly private system of care would almost certainly be lost in the resulting inflation.

NOTES

1. For the history of this debate, see Anderson, O. W., *The Uneasy Equilibrium: Private and Public Financing of Health Services in the United States, 1875-1965* (New Haven, Conn.: College and University Press, 1968).

2. For example, in 1967 the Harris Survey reported 51 percent of the population favored "a federal plan . . . such as Medicare . . . which would cover all members of your family." *The Washington Post*, Jan. 23, 1967.

3. Committee for National Health Insurance, Washington, D.C., *Health Security Program,* July 7, 1970.

4. *The Health of Americans,* Report of the 37th American Assembly (New York: Arden House, April 1970), p. 6.

5. For the 1970 version, see, for example, Roth, R. B., Medicredit—a national health services financing proposal. Paper prepared for National Health Forum, Washington, D.C., Feb. 1970. Also, periodic reports in *Amer. Med. News.*

6. Statement by Crosby, E. L., Sept. 8, 1969, Washington, D.C.

7. U.S. Department of Health, Education, and Welfare, Office of the Secretary, *Recommendations of the Task Force on Medicaid and Related Programs,* 1970, p. 93.

8. *New York Times,* Sept. 24, 1970.

9. These by no means exhaust the range of possibilities. Nothing has been said, for example, concerning a national health service along the British model. While such a development seems highly remote in terms of attitudes in the United States at the present time, there are a few authorities who believe it is the only viable solution for the long run. See, for example, E. Burns' discussion of "Beyond Medicare," *Amer. J. Public Health,* Apr. 1969, p. 619. While Mrs. Burns does not specifically call for an American national health service, her criticism of Dr. Isadore Falk's proposal in the same journal adds up to this conclusion.

10. Colman, J. D., Statement to Joint Legislative Committee on Problems of Public Health. New York City, Oct. 2, 1969, pp. 1-2.

11. Brown, R. E., Changing management and corporate structure. *Hospitals, J.A.H.A.,* Jan. 1, 1970, p. 83.

12. Pettengill, D. W., A program to improve the availability, acceptability, and financing of health care for all in the United States. Presented to U.S. House of Representatives, Committee on Ways and Means, Nov. 6, 1969, p. 10 ff.

13. United Hospital Fund of New York, *National Health Insurance: A Matter of Importance in the '70s,* 1970, pp. 10-24.

14. The Pettengill proposal does not quite fit this description. While it does provide benefit standards, participation is voluntary, administration is diffuse, and its state and federal subsidies would come entirely from general tax revenues. Under this scheme, however, most coverage would continue to be financed through private insurance and payroll deductions.

15. Somers, H. M. and A. R., *Workmen's Compensation: Prevention, Insurance, and Rehabilitation of Occupational Disability* (New York: Wiley, 1954), p. 123.

16. *New York Times,* Sept. 24, 1970.

17. Hearings before U.S. Senate, Committee on Finance, on H.R. 6675, April-May 1965, p. 459 ff.

18. National health insurance—problems and prospects. Michael M. Davis Lecture, University of Chicago, 1970, p. 24.

A Final Word

> What we are tackling in health care is probably one of the most complicated experiments in inter-governmental, inter-professional, and public-private relations ever undertaken in American history. . . . Moreover, we are tackling it at a time of resource constraints that make these hard choices much more difficult. The real test will come in the communities and the professions.
>
> IRVING J. LEWIS
> *New England Journal of Medicine* (October 16, 1969)

The four broad areas discussed in this book—health education, health manpower, the delivery system, and the financing mechanism—are all interrelated. Progress in any one area will be seriously impeded unless there is comparable progress in the others.

The money is there. The financing problem may well be the easiest to solve—if we can just devise a system that is adequate without being inflationary. We know, for example from FEP experience, that reasonably good coverage was being provided to some eight million persons in 1969 for a little over $100 per capita, about $400 per family (page 54). Virtually comprehensive coverage could have been provided in that year, through a combination of existing programs, for $224 to $285 per capita, or $733 to $851 per family.[1] These figures, computed by the Social Security Administration from rates charged by Group Health of Washington, D.C., one of the most expensive of all FEP carriers, Group Health Cooperative of Puget Sound, Washington, Group Health Dental Insurance of New York City, and a special HEW study of drug use,[2] include virtually complete hospitalization, physicians' services, dental care, and out-of-hospital prescribed drugs.

They do not include long-term mental illness or nursing home care. Even with these added, it seems clear that the nation's personal health care bill, as well as the overhead for research, professional education, public health services, and construction, could have been well met out of the $300 or so we spent per capita for these purposes in 1969. The tragedy is that while the money was spent most people were not getting anything like comprehensive care.

[1]For this and succeeding notes, see next page.

Obviously, to merely increase the flow of dollars will not itself provide a solution. Dollars can be a great lubricant for creaking social machinery and should be used as such. But a lubricant is not enough. There must be a sense of direction, a sense of purpose. The three other approaches to reform are indispensable.

The delivery system must be rationalized. The experience of the "socialized" European health care economies, which are going through many of the same difficulties as we are, including fast-rising costs and fragmentation of care, is proof that financial reforms alone are inadequate.[3] The concept of the franchised hospital, responsible for coordination of the full spectrum of comprehensive services to a defined community, appears to offer the most practical solution. Manpower, including physicians, must be increased substantially. Special attention must be paid to the development of primary physicians and physician-surrogates. New and more imaginative uses of the health care team, including the nurse and the druggist, must be developed and fitted into the evolving delivery system.

Perhaps most important of all, consumers must become better informed and more responsible as to the nature of health and illness and what they themselves can do to protect their own health. Without this, all else is likely to prove futile. As J. Douglas Colman has said, "We'll never get the job done, one patient at a time."[4]

We cannot know whether the medical care patterns of the future will excel ours. The only thing we know for sure is that they will be different. They can and should be better, in view of continuing scientific, educational, and economic progress. However, if the positive elements in the present trends do prevail, it will not be an automatic development, but will be because those who have a concern and a stake in our health care system—providers and consumers alike—take the trouble to understand the historical forces involved and deliberately seek to adapt themselves and their institutions to the new imperatives.

Discarding that which is obsolete or no longer relevant, emphasizing new forms of social and economic organization and new value systems to match the new science and technology, but always remaining true to the basic mission of the health professions—to promote health, heal the sick, rehabilitate the disabled, and comfort the dying—we can confront the current paradox of health care, with concern but without panic, in the spirit of Robert Browning, who saw the whole human enterprise as:

> . . . a paradox
> Which comforts while it mocks:
> Shall life succeed in that it seems to fail?

NOTES

1. Reed, L. S., and Carr, W. *The Benefit Structure of Private Health Insurance, 1968*, Research Report 32, U.S. Department of Health, Education, and Welfare, Social Security Administration, 1970, pp. 110-11.
2. *The Drug Users*, U.S. Department of Health, Education, and Welfare, Office of the Secretary, Task Force on Prescription Drugs, Background papers, 1968, pp. 20-22.
3. See, for example, Somers, A. R. The hospital is the core of the system. *Mod. Hosp.*, Sept. 1970, pp. 87-91.
4. Hilleboe Memorial Lecture, New York State Public Health Association, June 10, 1970, p. 8 (mimeo.).

EXCERPTS FROM "THE TRAGEDY OF THE COMMONS"

The following material was excerpted, with permission, from Garrett Hardin's "The Tragedy of the Commons," published in *Science* (Vol. 162, pp. 1243-48, December 13, 1968; copyright 1968 by the American Association for the Advancement of Science). Dr. Hardin's brilliant plea for the support of minimal but essential regulatory authority was advanced primarily on behalf of population control. It is equally applicable to the regulation of the health services industry.

We can make little progress . . . until we explicitly exorcise the spirit of Adam Smith. . . . In economic affairs, *The Wealth of Nations* (1776) popularized the "invisible hand," the idea than an individual who "intends only his own gain," is, at it were, "led by an invisible hand to promote . . . the public interest." Adam Smith did not assert that this was invariably true, and perhaps neither did any of his followers. But he contributed to a dominant tendency of thought that has ever since interfered with positive action based on rational analysis, namely, the tendency to assume that decisions reached individually will, in fact, be the best decisions for an entire society. If this assumption is correct it justifies the continuance of our present policy of laissez-faire. . . . If the assumption is not correct, we need to reexamine our individual freedoms to see which ones are defensible.

Tragedy of Freedom in a Commons

The rebuttal to the invisible hand . . . is to be found in a scenario first sketched in a little-known pamphlet in 1833 by a mathematical amateur named William Forster Lloyd (1794-1852). We may well call it "the tragedy of the commons," using the word "tragedy" as the philosopher Whitehead used it: "The essence of dramatic tragedy is not unhappiness. It resides in the solemnity of the remorseless working of things." He then goes on to say, "This inevitableness of destiny can only be illustrated in terms of human life by incidents which in fact involve unhappiness. For it is only by them that the futility of escape can be made evident in the drama."

The tragedy of the commons develops in this way. Picture a pasture open to all. It is to be expected that each herdsman will try to keep as many cattle as possible on the commons. Such an arrangement may work reasonably satisfactorily for centuries because tribal wars, poaching, and disease keep the numbers of both man and beast well below the carrying capacity of the land. Finally, however, comes the day of reckoning, that is, the day when the long-desired goal of social stability becomes a reality. At this point, the inherent logic of the commons remorselessly generates tragedy.

As a rational being, each herdsman seeks to maximize his gain. Explicitly or implicitly, more or less consciously, he asks, "What is the utility *to me* of adding one more animal to my herd?" This utility has one negative and one positive component.

1) The positive component is a function of the increment of one animal. Since the herdsman receives all the proceeds from the sale of the additional animal, the positive utility is nearly $+1$.

2) The negative component is a function of the additional overgrazing created by one more animal. Since, however, the effects of overgrazing are shared by all the herdsmen, the negative utility for any particular decision-making herdsman is only a fraction of -1.

Adding together the component partial utilities, the rational herdsman concludes that the only sensible course for him to pursue is to add another animal to his herd. And another; and another. . . . But this is the conclusion reached by each and every rational herdsman sharing a commons. Therein is the tragedy. Each man is locked into a system that compels him to increase his herd without limit—in a world that is limited. Ruin is the destination toward which all men rush, each pursuing his own best interest in a society that believes in the freedom of the commons. Freedom in a commons brings ruin to all.

Some would say that this is a platitude. Would that it were! In a sense, it was learned thousands of years ago, but natural selection favors the forces of psychological denial. The individual benefits as an individual from his ability to deny the truth even though society as a whole, of which he is a part, suffers. Education can counteract the natural tendency to do the wrong thing, but the inexorable succession of generations requires that the basis for this knowledge be constantly refreshed. . . .

In an approximate way, the logic of the commons has been understood for a long time, perhaps since the discovery of agriculture or the invention of private property in real estate. But it is understood mostly only in special cases which are not sufficiently generalized. Even at this late date, cattlemen leasing national land on the western ranges demonstrate no more than an ambivalent understanding, in constantly pressuring federal authorities to increase the head count to the point where overgrazing produces erosion and weed-dominance. Likewise, the oceans of the world continue to suffer from the survival of the philosophy of the commons. Maritime nations still respond automatically to the shibboleth of the "freedom of the seas." Professing to believe in the "inexhaustible resources of the oceans," they bring species after species of fish and whales closer to extinction. . . .

How To Legislate Temperance?

Analysis of the pollution problem as a function of population density uncovers a not generally recognized principle of morality, namely: *the morality of an act is a function of the state of the system at the time it is performed.* Using the commons as a cesspool does not harm the general public under frontier conditions, because there is no public; the same behavior in a metropolis is unbearable. A hundred and fifty years ago a plainsman could kill an American bison, cut out only the tongue for his dinner, and discard the rest of the animal. He was not in any important sense being wasteful. Today, with only a few thousand bison left, we would be appalled at such behavior. . . .

That morality is system-sensitive escaped the attention of most codifiers of ethics in the past. "Thou shalt not . . ." is the form of traditional ethical directives which make no allowance for particular circumstances. The laws of our society follow the pattern of ancient ethics, and therefore are poorly suited to governing a complex, crowded, changeable world. Our epicyclic solution is to augment statutory law with administrative law. Since it is practically impossible to spell out all the conditions under which it is safe to burn trash in the back yard or to run an automobile without smog-control, by law we delegate the details to bureaus. The result is administrative law, which is rightly feared for an ancient reason—*Quis custodiet ipsos custodes?*—"Who shall watch the watchers themselves?" John Adams said that we must have "a government of laws and not men." Bureau administrators, trying to evaluate the morality of acts in the total system, are singularly liable to corruption, producing a government by men, not laws.

Prohibition is easy to legislate (though not necessarily to enforce); but how do we legislate temperance? Experience indicates that it can be accomplished best through the mediation of administrative law. We limit possibilities unnecessarily if we suppose that the sentiment of *Quis custodiet* denies us the use of administrative law. We should rather retain the phrase as a perpetual reminder of fearful dangers we cannot avoid. The great challenge facing us now is to invent the corrective feedbacks that are needed to keep custodians honest. We must find ways to legitimate the needed authority of both the custodians and the corrective feedbacks. . . .

Pathogenic Effects of Conscience

If we ask a man who is exploiting a commons to desist "in the name of conscience," what are we saying to him? What does he hear?—not only at the moment but also in the wee small hours of the night when, half asleep, he remembers not merely the words we used but also the nonverbal communication cues we gave him unawares? Sooner or later, consciously or subconsciously, he senses that he has received two communications, and that they are contradictory: (i) (intended communication) "If you don't do as we ask, we will openly condemn you for not acting like a responsible citizen"; (ii) (the unintended communication) "If you *do* behave as we ask, we will secretly condemn you for a simpleton who can be shamed into standing aside while the rest of us exploit the commons."

Everyman then is caught in what Bateson has called a "double bind." Bateson and his co-workers have made a plausible case for viewing the double bind as an important causative factor in the genesis of schizophrenia. The double bind may not always be so damaging, but it always endangers the mental health of anyone to whom it is applied. "A bad conscience," said Nietzsche, "is a kind of illness."

To conjure up a conscience in others is tempting to anyone who wishes to extend his control beyond the legal limits. Leaders at the highest level succumb to this temptation. Has any President during the past generation failed to call on labor unions to moderate voluntarily their demands for higher wages, or to steel companies to honor voluntary guidelines on prices? I can recall none. The rhetoric used on such occasions is designed to produce feelings of guilt in noncooperators.

For centuries it was assumed without proof that guilt was a valuable, perhaps even an indispensable, ingredient of the civilized life. Now, in this post-Freudian world, we doubt it.

Paul Goodman speaks from the modern point of view when he says: "No good has ever come from feeling guilty, neither intelligence, policy, nor compassion. The guilty do not pay attention to the object but only to themselves, and not even to their own interests, which might make sense, but to their anxieties. . . ."

Mutual Coercion Mutually Agreed Upon

If the word responsibility is to be used at all, I suggest that it be in the sense Charles Frankel uses it. "Responsibility," says this philosopher, "is the product of definite social arrangements." Notice that Frankel calls for social arrangements—not propaganda.

The social arrangements that produce responsibility are arrangements that create coercion, of some sort. Consider bank-robbing. The man who takes money from a bank acts as if the bank were a commons. How do we prevent such action? Certainly not by trying to control his behavior solely by a verbal appeal to his sense of responsibility. Rather than rely on propaganda we follow Frankel's lead and insist that a bank is not a commons; we seek the definite social arrangements that will keep it from becoming a commons. That we thereby infringe on the freedom of would-be robbers we neither deny nor regret.

The morality of bank-robbing is particularly easy to understand because we accept complete prohibition of this activity. We are willing to say "Thou shalt not rob banks," without providing for exceptions. But temperance also can be created by coercion. Taxing is a good coercive device. To keep downtown shoppers temperate in their use of parking space we introduce parking meters for short periods, and traffic fines for longer ones. We need not actually forbid a citizen to park as long as he wants to; we need merely make it increasingly expensive for him to do so. Not prohibition, but carefully biased options are what we offer him. A Madison Avenue man might call this persuasion; I prefer the greater candor of the word coercion.

Coercion is a dirty word to most liberals now, but it need not forever be so. As with the four-letter words, its dirtiness can be cleansed away by exposure to the light, by saying it over and over without apology or embarrassment. To many, the word coercion implies arbitrary decisions of distant and irresponsible bureaucrats; but this is not a necessary part of its meaning. The only kind of coercion I recommend is mutual coercion, mutually agreed upon by the majority of the people affected. To say that we mutually agree to coercion is not to say that we are required to enjoy it, or even to pretend we enjoy it. Who enjoys taxes? We all grumble about them. But we accept compulsory taxes because we recognize that voluntary taxes would favor the conscienceless. We institute and (grumblingly) support taxes and other coercive devices to escape the horror of the commons. . . .

It is one of the peculiarities of the warfare between reform and the status quo that it is thoughtlessly governed by a double standard. Whenever a reform measure is proposed it is often defeated when its opponents triumphantly discover a flaw in it. As Kingsley Davis has pointed out, worshippers of the status quo sometimes imply that no reform is possible without unanimous agreement, an implication contrary to historical fact. As nearly as I can make out, automatic rejection of proposed reforms is based on one of two unconscious assumptions: (i) that the status quo is perfect; or (ii) that the choice we face is between reform and no action; if the proposed reform is imperfect, we presumably should take no action at all, while we wait for a perfect proposal.

But we can never do nothing. That which we have done for thousands of years is also action. It also produces evils. Once we are aware that status quo is action, we can then compare its discoverable advantages and disadvantages with the predicted advantages and disadvantages of the proposed reform, discounting as best we can for our lack of experience. On the basis of such a comparison, we can make a rational decision which will not involve the unworkable assumption that only perfect systems are tolerable.

Recognition of Necessity

Perhaps the simplest summary of this analysis . . . is this: the commons, if justifiable at all, is justifiable only under conditions of low-population density. As the human population has increased, the commons has had to be abandoned in one aspect after another.

First we abandoned the commons in food gathering, enclosing farm land and restricting pastures and hunting and fishing areas. These restrictions are still not complete throughout the world.

Somewhat later we saw that the commons as a place for waste disposal would also have to be abandoned. Restrictions on the disposal of domestic sewage are widely accepted in the Western world; we are still struggling to close the commons to pollution by automobiles, factories, insecticide sprayers, fertilizing operations, and atomic energy installations.

In a still more embryonic state is our recognition of the evils of the commons in matters of pleasure. There is almost no restriction on the propagation of sound waves in the public medium. The shopping public is assaulted with mindless music, without its consent. Our government is paying out billions of dollars to create supersonic transport which will disturb 50,000 people for every one person who is whisked from coast to coast 3 hours faster. Advertisers muddy the airwaves of radio and television and pollute the view of travelers. We are a long way from outlawing the commons in matters of pleasure. Is this because our Puritan inheritance makes us view pleasure as something of a sin, and pain (that is, the pollution of advertising) as the sign of virtue?

Every new enclosure of the commons involves the infringement of somebody's personal liberty. Infringements made in the distant past are accepted because no contemporary complains of a loss. It is the newly proposed infringements that we vigorously oppose; cries of "rights" and "freedom" fill the air. But what does "freedom" mean? When men mutually agreed to pass laws against robbing, mankind became more free, not less so. Individuals locked into the logic of the commons are free only to bring on universal ruin; once they see the necessity of mutual coercion, they become free to pursue other goals. I believe it was Hegel who said, "Freedom is the recognition of necessity."

Appendix B

SPECIFIC ISSUES FOR INVESTIGATION IN RELATION TO ANY PROPOSED NATIONAL HEALTH INSURANCE PROGRAM

> This material was excerpted from the Department of Health, Education, and Welfare's *Report of the Task Force on Medicaid and Related Programs,* "Long-Term Financing Policies," June 1970.

Delineation of objectives is necessary to establish broad goals and direction. To determine whether particular policies or plans are likely to move us toward such goals, in what degree and over what period of time, requires answers to numerous specific questions.

In this section we attempt to spell out some of the issues and questions that must be raised in respect to any plan or policy that is to be seriously considered in order to anticipate its likely consequences and to weigh the comparative advantages and disadvantages of different policies. Positive knowledge or empirical data are not available to offer definitive answers to many important questions. Nevertheless, such questions must be raised and the best available thought and experience directed at finding the most reasonable answers possible. The issues and questions demonstrate the enormous complexity and vast range of the issues that must be considered. They indicate that Government policy relates not only to its own programs but affects the organization, financing, and delivery of care throughout the health economy.

The sheer magnitude and diversity of problems suggest that while coherent public policy is called for there is unlikely to be a single all-embracing solution. No one program can win all pluses and no minuses among the issues to be resolved. The proposed study will have to think in terms of trade-offs and compromises, giving something up here in order to gain something there. If we are not to incur excessive rigidity, we probably will have to plan in terms of a variety of policies that are rationally interrelated and mutually supportive within a defined set of public goals, unified but not unitary.

The issues and questions are listed under four broad categories: financing, administration, resource capacity, and demand. Many of these cut across two or more of these categories. Thus, frequently, the location of a particular question proves arbitrary; this should not be interpreted as an attempt to confine its consideration any more narrowly than the question warrants.

A. *Financing*

  1. Techniques should be developed for careful calculation of probable initial and projected costs—both public and private—of proposed programs.

159

2. Because different programs propose quite different benefit packages, any estimate of costs should be related to the kinds of services to be covered and the extent to which such services will be used.

3. All serious proposals will require revenues of dimensions that will have significant economic and political influences. Such proposals include financing through general revenues, payroll deductions, and direct consumer payments in varying forms and mixes. Attempts should be made to weigh the probable effects of the various revenue-raising schemes, as well as the totals to be raised, upon:

   — the efficacy of the program itself, including prices of services;

   — administrative costs and complexities;

   — the general economy;

   — public finance:

   • over-all tax structure;

   • budgetary and fiscal implications of huge transfer of funds from private to public sector; and

   • extent to which the necessary tax increase may affect work and production incentives; and

   — political and popular acceptability.

4. With the growth of social insurance, there has been a great deal of discussion about the regressiveness of payroll taxes (or, at least, that portion paid by employees). In the social security program, this is largely offset by a progressive benefit structure. Are similar offsets contemplated in the proposed plans? Any proposed system of financing health care will involve some redistribution of income. How extensive should the redistribution be? Does dependence on a single source of revenue jeopardize the financing mechanism?

5. Despite the relative progressiveness of general-revenue taxes, it is recognized that the increasing demands on public finance in modern society require a wide diversity of revenue-producing devices. Payroll taxes have been widely accepted as peculiarly appropriate for social insurance, not only because they relieve what might otherwise appear as an inordinate strain on general revenues, but because of the visible financial and psychological connection between revenues and benefits. Leaving aside the academic dispute as to whether social insurance is or is not "real" insurance, the psychological advantages of relating personal benefits to "earned rights" or "paid-for rights" are often stressed. What is the applicability of such considerations to a health program? What is the role of earmarked payroll taxes?

6. Direct consumer payments are in varying degrees and forms included in virtually all proposals, and are intended either to limit the program's liability or costs or to act as restraints upon unwarranted consumption.

The relative progressiveness or regressiveness of such payments deserve the same examination as the formal tax aspects. What is the appropriate role, if any, for deductibles, coinsurance and maximums? Should they be income-related?

7. All proposals assume in varying degrees the continuation of private financing of the health economy. Should private financing be regarded as merely an unavoidable appendage, or are there potential advantages in a public-private mix that should be consciously explored and promoted? Are some aspects of the private-market economy necessary or useful for guidelines, restraints, disciplines, or stimulants to the public program?

8. Is a noncompulsory public system, even if largely Government subsidized (as in the various tax-credit schemes) likely to achieve its coverage objectives? Which groups in the population are likely to respond to the subsidies and which are not, i.e., youth, the poor, the chronically ill?

9. All proposals assume some degree of personal payments or contributions for health care. What happens to the poor who cannot make these payments? What are the sources of funds to meet this need and how should they be channeled? Attempts should be made to measure the continuing burden on public assistance for health care under each major proposal. What are the implications of this burden?

B. *Administration*

1. Important issues for administrative organization, as well as financing, are the desirable mix of public and private instrumentalities—profit and non-profit—and centralization vs. decentralization. Almost all protagonists have indicated awareness of dangers in a single monolithic program, dangers of rigidity and sluggish responsiveness to change; all current plans thus claim to have elements of decentralization intended to avoid or minimize such dangers. The public-private question may be considered under several broad questions:

   — What is the appropriate role of private agencies in a publicly mandated program?

   — What is the appropriate role of private instrumentalities independent of the public program?

   — What is the appropriate structure of the private instrumentality—profit or nonprofit?

2. Some plans propose direct Government subsidies for insurance to be bought from private underwriters; others propose complete mixes of compulsory Government financing with private underwriting and benefit management.

   — If there were to be a relatively comprehensive, mandated Governmental health-insurance plan:

     • Is it more desirable that the existing private health-insurance apparatus be dismantled or that their skills and experience be harnessed for the public program to serve as intermediaries as in Medicare, as agents of Government under management contracts, or as competitive under-writers as in the FEHB?

- Would decentralized administration be meaningful in terms of policy initiatives, varieties of program patterns, etc.?

- In considering the use of private organizations in administration and of centralization vs. decentralization, what account should be taken of the size of the Federal bureaucracy that would be required? What would be the problem of developing adequate technical competence for this complex field in 50 State bureaucracies if responsibility were to be delegated to that level?

— If there were to be a "mixed" program (of Javits or FEHB type) or a tax-credit program (AMA), should the present multitude of carriers be free to participate, or does such Government financing suggest the need for limitation of number and types of carriers so that advantage may be taken of economies of scale, efficiency, and ease of Government control and communication?

— Under which approach would innovation be more likely?

In such inquiries the experience of Medicare and the FEHB program should be instructive and, therefore, closely examined.

3. Under any scheme, there inevitably will continue to exist health expenditures not subsidized nor mandated by Government. Should not the size, character, and role of the expenditures to be met from private sources be considered simultaneously with the planning of the public program?

— In a controlled public program, even if decentralized in operation, can there be sufficient incentives for venturesomeness, for risk-taking innovation . . . and at what cost? Can the radically unorthodox challenge prove viable within the context of a national public program?

— If not, or if not sufficiently so, should the public program contemplate such a role for the private sector . . . perhaps encourage it?

— The great bulk of American higher education takes place in public institutions. But, it is generally agreed that the standards and relative political independence of the public institutions have been substantially protected by the continued vitality of strong private institutions (illustrated, for example, during the McCarthyism era). Are there parallels to be drawn for the health field?

4. One desirable quality of a new, untried program is that in its early years, at least, it be framed to provide maximum flexibility and maneuverability to be restructured, and a minimum number of features from which there can be virtually no retreat. How do the different proposals compare on this score?

5. If Government were to be the major purchaser of services, what are the implications for privately-owned, privately-operated institutions—hospitals and extended care facilities?

— Are there regulatory devices and controls that would prove effective to assure public accountability?

— To what extent is ownership or governorship by Government necessary or inevitable?

6. If either publicly- or privately-insured medical benefits, alone or in combination, account for a preponderance of physicians' services, can market controls be assumed to apply in the sense of favorably affecting price? If not, what types of controls might be needed?

7. If the Federal Government is to assume financial and other responsibility for a health program, is this compatible with the system of individual State licensing of practitioners and health institutions and with other State laws that may restrict the program (such as the illegality of prepaid group-practice plans in some states)? Will the entire Federal law-making and regulatory role in the health field require reconsideration?

8. In plans involving primarily Federal subsidy of private insurance, what new kind and degree of regulation of insurance may be required? Prices? Profit margins? Benefit packages? Is continuation of State regulation feasible under such conditions? Will uniform Federal regulation be necessary?

9. How can we avoid the familiar danger of stimulating public expectations that cannot, in practice, be fully satisfied? Is it better to concentrate responsibility for problems of so broad a scope and political sensitivity on one administrative agency or to "spread the heat" among a number of institutions? Which of these arrangements is likely to prove more accessible and responsive to public demand or protest?

C. *Resource Capacity*

1. Can demand for services under various proposals be projected in order to determine what resources are needed?

2. To the extent that demand can be estimated, can the adequacy of resource capacity be projected?

— By categories of service?

— By geographic area?

3. Does the program make adequate provision for capital needed to maintain supply resources in terms of facilities and manpower?

— What are the sources for capital funding? What are the other alternatives —for example, an allowance in operating expenses or by appropriation— to a reimbursement formula?

— How could a meaningful role for private philanthropy be maintained and encouraged?

4. Since such public funding is inevitably restricted, will not short supply cause increased opting for services outside the public system by upper and middle classes as has happened in other countries? What are the implications for relative access by the poor? Is there a way of assuring that the private sector will augment resources, not just draw upon existing supply?

5. What alternative public policies could stimulate the private sector to augment the current resource capacity and not just draw upon existing supply?

— Long lead time from passage of legislation to date of implementation? How long? What can be done in interim?

— Implementation by gradual stages within certain populations to be covered: e.g., initially, children to age 14; subsequently, ages 45-64; a few years later, the remaining population?

— Implementation by gradual stages in range of services to be covered?

— Movement into full program promptly on theory that only effective demand can force an adequate and appropriate supply response, and that the temporary dislocations are worth the price in long-run terms?

6. There is widespread agreement that significant changes in the delivery system are needed. Many people believe that only a massive insurance program can induce needed change. Others fear that such a program—even accompanied by regulation—is more likely to preserve the present system without changing its structure by the sheer fact of financially underpinning it. How can this be avoided? Are grants for experimentation enough to produce change in the system? Is there sufficient incentive in the grant mechanism to stimulate innovative change? Could the method of approving requests for grants be altered in a way that would allow support for innovative experiments? Do we know how to facilitate change other than by building in some competition? How can this be done in a public system? Does this suggest some planned role for the private sector?

7. With vast new purchasing power thrown into the system, will extraordinary inflation result in constriction of supply? How is this to be avoided?

D. *Demand*

1. Experience of other nations suggests that the potential demand for health services may be virtually boundless if left entirely to find its own level. The dramatic advances in medical science and technological capacities—e.g., transplants, implantations of artificial organs, dialysis, and the many other "miracles" waiting in the wings—underscore the point. Are restraints on demand essential? How is this to be done? Who is to make the decision?

— Direct restraint on demand? What kind? By whom?

— Indirect restraint on demand by limiting or controlling supply?

— Is some type of deliberate rationing called for? What kind?

2. How effective are deductibles, copayment, coinsurance and indemnity in containing demand?

   — At what point may they result in undesirable under-utilization?

   — Do they restrict demand mainly of poor and near-poor?

   — Are they worth the burden in administrative and other costs?

3. If restrictions are used, should they favor short-term or long-term care? Should there be emphasis on early, preventive care? Or, on meeting catastrophic needs?

4. If demand is to be controlled by setting deliberate limits on available supply, what guides, if any, are available (for example, through areawide planning) for rational decision making?

5. What incentives or controls may be feasible and adequate to cause providers to contain potential demand?

   — Use of lowest cost levels of appropriate care?

   — Minimizing laboratory and x-ray procedures?

   — Relating volume of routine physical checkups to cost-benefit considerations?

   — Utilization review?

   — Areawide planning?

   — Consumer education?

   — Systems for improved records on patient care?

6. Should there be a conscious policy of directing certain types of demand to the privately financed sector? How should these be selected?

Index